Dr. Khem Shahani truly is the Father of today's probiotic industry. His research and products have helped my clients for over twenty years. Probiotics build health; overuse of antibiotics in animal feed and in "people medicine" eventually destroys health. This book is a "must read" for every health professional and the patients they serve.

Bonnie C. Minsky, MA, MPH, CNS, LDN, Public Health Educator
Author of *Nutrition in a Nutshell* and *Our Children's Health*

Dr. Shahani's essential guide to probiotics is the first book on friendly bacteria that I can recommend wholeheartedly to thousands of professional athletes and doctors who trust in our nutritional advice. If this book would be read and its recommendations followed by everyone, we would have much less sickness in the world and a lot more optimal performance.

Douglas Grant, Optimal Health Systems President
NBA Nutritionist

When I was growing up my Dad, a dentist, used to take jars of my mother's homemade yogurt to his patients who were on antibiotics. This simple introduction of helpful bacteria prevented all manner of side effects. I have carried on my father's wise practice for 25 years in my work in women's health. I consider probiotics one of the most useful—and underutilized—modalities available for preserving health.

This book is an outstanding guide to a critically important health topic!

Christiane Northrup, M.D.
Author of NY Times bestsellers, *Women's Bodies, Women's Wisdom*
and *The Wisdom of Menopause and Mother-Daughter Wisdom:
Creating a Legacy of Physical and Emotional Health*

Everyone who is serious about the relationship of microflora to health should read this book. The professor's unique view and extremely broad, inclusive approach to probiotics and health provides an insight into maladies commonly relegated to a narrow view of medicine. This publication is timely and essential to professionals in biochemistry, microbiology, and nutrition, as well as those seeking to understand how science is done in the uncertain world of supplements. Dr. Shahani has truly performed a service to mankind's children through his dedication to this work.

Paul J. Whalen, B.S., M.S. (microbiology), Ph.D. (food technology)

Note: Dr. Whalen is a prominent food research scientist in the U.S. food industry. He studied under Dr. Shahani at the University of Nebraska-Lincoln for his doctorate.

# DEDICATION

*To Mankind's Children,*
*The Inheritors*
*of the Future*

# CULTIVATE HEALTH FROM WITHIN

## DR. SHAHANI'S GUIDE TO PROBIOTICS

Khem M. Shahani, Ph.D.

with

Betsy F. Meshbesher, D.C.

Venkat Mangalampalli, Ph.D.

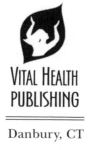

VITAL HEALTH
PUBLISHING

Danbury, CT

# CONTENTS

———————◆———————

THE UNITED NATIONS
WORLD HEALTH ORGANIZATION (WHO)
has asked doctors to create a "New Medicine,"
calling for a rebirth of ancient medical traditions.
It urged governments to give "adequate importance
to the utilization of their traditional systems of medicine."
(from resolution WHA30.49).

———————◆———————

*Nature created her cures in a safe and balanced way. It is our personal hope that this guide may contribute to the movement that is in the direction of the above important WHO call. Thank you for your interest in health and this mutual concern we share.*

Dr. Khem M. Shahani
Dr. Betsy F. Meshbesher
Dr. Venkat Mangalampalli

# FOREWORD
## by Frederic J. Vagnini, M.D., FACS, FACN

I am honored and humbled to write this introduction. I feel that *Cultivate Health From Within: Dr. Shahani's Guide to Probiotics* covers an extremely important aspect of medicine, health, and longevity. It is special because the work of Dr. Khem Shahani, particularly with the DDS-1 strain of *Lactobacillus acidophilus*, which he developed and named, places him in a distinguished class achieved by very few scientists. His many years of research, clinical results, and findings leave a legacy of inspiration and good health for millions of individuals worldwide.

This book, presented in a simple and concise form, should be part of all medical students' curriculum, as well as required reading for all healthcare professionals. I personally feel that the importance of the probiotic story needs to be embraced by health care givers around the world.

Has 21st-century medicine overlooked the importance of a simple health management system? With heart transplants, robotic surgery, hi-tech computer diagnostics, gene therapy, modern drugs, and cell engineering all in widespread use, the obvious basic health management systems are being ignored. This is why complimentary or holistic medicine is extremely important. Holistic practitioners have realized that lifestyle changes are the keys to good health and a long life. This is especially important since poor diet, lack of exercise, and stress are the leading causes of aging and health deterioration. Today's diet is too frequently high in saturated fats, trans fats, chemicals, food additives, toxins, and simple sugars. This diet, along with the stress factors of living in a highly technological world, has introduced an epidemic of intestinal dysbiosis. (Dysbiosis refers to the condition where the normal healthy population of beneficial bacteria in the intestines has been disrupted, leaving it open to the overgrowth of yeast, fungi, parasites, and potentially harmful strains of bacteria. This intestinal imbalance in turn adversely affects other important organ systems via toxic stress and interfering with nutrient absorption and utilization). I believe that intestinal dysbiosis is the precursor to general health deterioration and a multitude of symptoms—even multiple organ failure. Symptoms very frequently include fatigue, arthritis, brain fog, weight gain, and "just not feeling well."

In my health centers in New York, which deal with cardiovascular disease, obesity, and diabetes, the majority of patients I see for any type of problem have a common complaint: "I just do not feel well" or "I am tired." They have impaired intestinal health with various symptoms including constipation, gas, bloating, diarrhea, and acid reflux. Because of these common complaints from my heart patients, I became interested in intestinal health—I believe in the total management of the patient. Probiotics have now become a part of my standard treatment protocol, along with lifestyle and dietary changes.

The history of probiotics, especially from a clinician's point of view, has changed over the years. When I first started doing clinical nutrition some 25 years ago, even as I was a cardiovascular surgeon, it became apparent that most physicians ignored the Candida connection (yeast overgrowth). Many relegated yeast to gynecology. Even today, there is little realization that a multitude of symptoms, including gas, indigestion, bloating, irritable bowel, constipation, diarrhea, as well as fatigue, arthritis, muscle aches, and brain fog, are related to systemic yeast infections. Continued education in the medical field and to the general public will be necessary to help people with these problems.

Today, many doctors are not even aware of the fact that Candida antibodies can be detected with a simple blood test and a stool culture. Very few will know how to treat it if indeed there is Candida overgrowth cultured from the stool.

Since many healthcare professionals are not even aware that there is such a thing as the yeast connection or intestinal dysbiosis, they have difficulty ordering proper tests and diagnosing the problem. Even in cases where a decision has been made to treat the dysbiosis, proper diet is not used; the right intestinal support nutrients are not used; food allergies are not removed; and lifestyle changes, including diet and exercise, are underutilized. This book illustrates the importance of diagnosing, preventing, and treating intestinal dysbiosis, and of choosing the right probiotic strains to help overcome the associated health issues.

There is little doubt that there is a connection between the 21st-century diabetes/obesity epidemic and the fact that cardiovascular disease, including heart attack and stroke, is still the number one killer in the United States. Diabetes has now been reclassified by the American Diabetes Association not only as an endocrine disease but also a cardiovascular disease. The new explosion in the medical literature reporting on the Metabolic Syndrome, or Syndrome X or hyperinsulinemia, further elucidates the heart disease/ diabetes/insulin/obesity connection. How does this all relate to probiotics? The answer is simple. I have seen thousands of patients who reveal the so-called insulin-heart disease connection. In addition to their cardiovascular symptoms they almost all have gastrointestinal symptoms. The causes are often related to food allergies, chemicals, artificial sweeteners, excessive saturated and trans fats, and poor food choices like excessive simple sugars and low-nutrient foods. Most of these patients have intestinal dysbiosis and the resulting impaired gut permeability. The proper lifestyle changes along with probiotic supplementation are an important component in my patient care. I have found that managing the gut symptoms in the cardiovascular patients improves their general health, improves immunity, gives more energy, helps control glucose/insulin levels, and promotes weight loss.

Recent medical literature has been reporting on the new area of *inflammation* as an etiologic agent for disease. At a recent meeting of the American Academy of Anti-Aging Medicine, the theme was inflammation. It is now apparent that most degenerative diseases have an inflammatory component. Certainly, heart disease and arteriosclerosis appear to be intensified by inflammation. This has been proved by epidemiological studies and evaluating high-sensitivity C-reactive protein (Hi-CRP). The research relating higher C-reactive protein levels and greater incidence of cardiovascular disease is clear and quite conclusive. Diabetes and obesity are also considered inflammatory diseases. Information from two studies on the statin trials indicated that lower CRP levels are associated with fewer cardiovascular events independent of LDL cholesterol levels. Their studies were reported in the January 6, 2005 *New England Journal of Medicine.*

As I noted above, my clinical practice has identified many heart patients with associated obesity and hyperinsulinemia, most of whom have associated GI problems. Diabetes, obesity, arthritis, neurodegenerative disease, eye disorders, and many other medical problems, including skin diseases, have been related to inflammation. Since the use of probiotics will improve GI function *and* improve the inflammatory cascade problem, probiotic supplementation should be a part of the treatment management of all GI, inflammatory, and hyperinsulinemia problems. This will help overall health and decrease the progression of degenerative disease.

Modern research continues to realize the importance of probiotic research. With the explosion of "baby boomers" reaching middle age and older, there has been an increasing interest in anti-aging therapies. This has opened up an entirely new field of probiotic application: utilizing probiotics' well-documented but little-realized immuno-enhancing properties. Hopefully, this book will serve to educate the medical field and the public about the important role of probiotics in health, and allow Dr. Shahani's legacy to help millions of individuals for many years to come.

Dr. Frederic J. Vagnini is unique among physicians and health educators worldwide. After graduation from St. Louis University School of Medicine in 1963, Dr. Vagnini spent eight years in post-doctorate internship and residency, studying surgery (vascular, heart, and lung surgery) at the Downstate Medical Center, Brooklyn, New York, and at Columbia Presbyterian Medical Center, New York, New York. Upon completion of this training, Dr. Vagnini served in the United States Army as a Lieutenant Colonel and subsequently entered private practice on Long Island, New York. For the next 25 years Dr. Vagnini practiced as a heart, lung, and blood-vessel surgeon, operating on thousands of patients with heart and vascular disease. During the course of his career, Dr. Vagnini became interested in Health Education, Preventive Medicine, and Clinical Nutrition. Because of his vast experience in the area of heart disease and nutrition, he became a frequent guest speaker and has appeared numerous times on local and national radio and television.

In the print area of Health Education, Dr. Vagnini has written hundreds of articles in the lay literature and for numerous scientific publications. He also publishes a monthly newsletter, "Cardiovascular Wellness Newsletter." This publication covers current health news issues, with appropriate commentary.

Dr. Vagnini is certified by the American Board of Surgery and the American Board of Thoracic Surgery. He is an active, highly respected member of numerous medical societies, including:

The American College of Surgeons (Fellow)

The American Society of Echocardiography

The American College of Chest Physicians (Fellow)

The American College of Nutrition (Fellow)

The Holistic Medical Society

The American Medical Association (AMA)

The American Association of Clinical Nutritionists

The Nassau County Medical Society

The American Heart Association

The Presbyterian Hospital Alumni

The National Stroke Association

The Nassau Surgical Society

The International Society for Free Radical Research

The New York Cardiological Society

The New York Society for Thoracic Surgery

The American Association of Diabetes Educators

The American College of Cardiology (Fellow)

The International Academy of Nutrition and Preventive Medicine

The American Society for Surgical Research (Fellow)

The American Society of Hypertension

The American College of Angiology (Fellow)

The American Society of Bariatric Physicians

# FOREWORD
## by Ramesh Chandan, Ph.D.

As a former graduate student and research associate of Dr. Khem Shahani, I am very impressed by the way he and his coauthors, Dr. Betsy F. Meshbesher and Dr. Venkat Mangalampalli, have communicated the complex subject of probiotics and their efficacy to the consumer in *Cultivate Health from Within*. Dr. Shahani was truly a pioneer in conducting sound scientific studies on the beneficial health attributes of consuming *Lactobacillus acidophilus*, other lactobacilli, and bifidobacteria. For over forty years, Dr. Shahani's laboratory published dozens of original research articles on the health attributes of probiotics. This research work was so original, and the results were so unique, that the University of Nebraska–Lincoln, as well as Dr. Shahani himself, received recognition and prestige in the form of numerous awards from scientific organizations around the world.

Dr. Shahani's work elucidated how yogurt culture helps in the digestion of lactose in lactose-intolerant individuals. His research showed reduction of serum cholesterol as a result of consumption of acidophilus products. He and his coworkers demonstrated immune-system enhancement by consumption of probiotic cultures, including the specific strain *Lactobacillus acidophilus* DDS-1 and bifidobacteria. He found that all probiotic dietary adjuncts do not possess the same viability and the same beneficial value. He devised technologies to enhance the viability and stability of *Lactobacillus acidophilus* DDS-1 and other probiotics under various storage conditions. In order to make these unique and viable strains available to the consumer, he established Nebraska Cultures as a high-quality probiotics manufacturer.

Prior to Dr. Shahani's research findings, the scientific and medical community did not generally recognize the health merits of probiotic cultures. With the help of Dr. Shahani's research, compelling data made a profound impact on the philosophy of health maintenance and improvement. The results of his probiotics research convinced many clinicians around the world of these outstanding health benefits. In this regard, Dr. Shahani initiated a movement to bring the science of probiotics and their use directly to consumers concerned with improving their health.

Besides generating scientific data on the health benefits of consuming probiotics, Dr. Shahani was a great communicator among healthcare professionals and the medical community. He lectured tirelessly on this subject to numerous groups around the world. During these years of speaking engagements, he felt there was a need to develop a book that would explain various aspects of probiotics to the consumer. This book fulfills his dream of addressing the questions and concerns of consumers in easily understood language. Dr. Meshbesher and Dr. Manglapalli have been associated with Dr. Shahani for many years and have brought a wealth of their experience to the book.

In reviewing the book, I found it very informative, based on research data and contemporary thought. The book is easy to read, and it thoroughly comprehends the complex area of probiotics. Interest in this area of research has brought forth mounting evidence for the health benefits of using probiotics in the form of supplements or as components of foods. It is exciting that this book is being published so that consumers can understand and benefit from the role of probiotics in everyday life.

# Introduction to the Gastrointestinal System

## *The "Gut" Feeling*

**GUT** [from Old English *geotan*, to pour]: *All or part of the food pipe which passes through the body, including the stomach and the intestine.*[1,2]

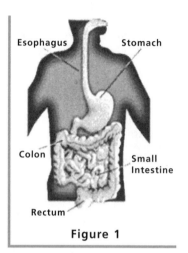

Esophagus  Stomach

Colon  Small Intestine

Rectum

**Figure 1**

Each and every person naturally has billions of microorganisms living in their gastrointestinal system—more popularly known as "the gut." In fact, there are more bacteria in one human body than there are numbers of people in the world. These bacteria are essential to the normal function of both our gastrointestinal and immune systems.

There are more than 400 different types of bacterial species that live in the human gut (six major groups and many other minor groups). Incredibly, this amounts to $3^{1}/_{2}$ pounds of bacteria in the intestines at all times, several thousand billion in each person (more than all the cells in a human body). About one-third of the fecal matter which you pass (water removed) consists of bacteria. Fortunately, less than 1 percent of all known types of microorganisms are undesirable or pathogenic. Yet that 1 percent can multiply into overwhelming numbers, defeat the friendly microorganisms, take over the territory, and cause anything from mild distress to virulent disease and death.

Though appearing as a system "within" the human body, the gastrointestinal tract is actually a tube that is continual, with the external environment at both ends: mouth and anus. This open tube is filled with a mixture of food particles (in various stages of digestion) and solid waste particles.

---

### EXTERNAL FACTORS
#### AFFECTING THE GASTROINTESTINAL SYSTEM

Those factors which exist outside the GI system—
beyond the mouth and anus.

*Examples:*
1. Individuals and the structures and forces that make up the outer environment.
2. The types of food and supplements available from the outer world.
3. The toxins and chemicals in the outer world.
4. The microorganisms living in the outer world.

**Figure 2: FACTORS THAT AFFECT THE GI SYSTEM**

---

Figure 1 illustrates the gastrointestinal system (GI system), with its major parts labeled. Each part is adapted for a specific function that contributes to the overall function of the entire system. The ability of the GI system to optimally perform is related to numerous factors. These can be divided into two major categories: external factors and internal factors (Figure 2).

The job of the gastrointestinal system is to break down bulk food, absorb essential nutrients, and then provide the body with a continual supply of them for its normal function, maintenance, and repair. The system must simultaneously provide continual elimination of the useless waste.

Normally, food is digested partially in the mouth and stomach. In the intestine, the partially digested food is ultimately metabolized by the millions and millions of "good guy" microorganisms working simultaneously and synergistically.

If we eat the wrong kinds and amounts of food, the "bad guy" undesirable or pathogenic bacteria will feed on these food stuffs and produce toxins that will be absorbed into the bloodstream. Known as intestinal toxemia, it reflects one concept of disease: We can literally poison ourselves by way of our intestinal tract.

Hence, good health depends on the maintenance of proper intestinal flora. A healthy intestine is one that maintains a critical balance between various groups of these bacteria. Any suboptimal or unhealthy condition (stress, onset of disease, ingestion of

## INTERNAL FACTORS
### AFFECTING THE GASTROINTESTINAL SYSTEM

Those factors which are already inside the GI system—located somewhere between the mouth and anus.

*Examples:*
1. The actual cells, tissues, and organs that make up the structure of the GI system.
2. The types of food and supplements that have entered the GI system.
3. The transient buildup of toxins and chemicals (including drugs) and waste in the GI system.
4. The microorganisms that have somehow entered and now live in the GI system.

**FACTORS THAT AFFECT THE GI SYSTEM (cont.)**

antibiotics and/or medicines, alcohol or nicotine abuse, improper food or rest) or other harmful environmental conditions, including chronic exposure to potential toxins (heavy metals, for instance), may endanger this balance in the intestinal flora, resulting in the reduction of the friendly or beneficial bacteria, such as lactobacilli.

Since there are many conditions that can disturb the balance of a normal gastrointestinal system, it is the responsibility of our nervous system (Figure 3) to alert us to any problems in the GI system. The nervous system (with help from the hormonal system) also regulates gastrointestinal activity.

Many activities of the nervous system are initiated by sensory experience coming from sensory receptors on the surface of the body or in body cells, tissues, or organs. The nervous system would not be at all effective in controlling bodily functions if each bit of sensory information caused a reaction. Therefore, one of the major functions of the nervous system is to process incoming information in such a way that appropriate responses (involuntary and voluntary) occur.

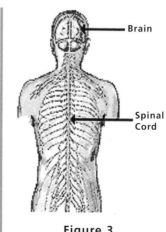

Figure 3

Indeed, more than 99 percent of all sensory information is discarded by the brain as irrelevant and unimportant. After the important sensory information has been selected, it is then channeled into specific regions of the brain to generate specific responses.[3] Sufficient *imbalance* in the gastrointestinal system can create a displeasing sensation, whereas sufficient *balance* sustains that easy "all is right" sensation.

Crucial for keeping that healthy "gut feeling" is a constantly maintained, healthy gastrointestinal microecology—bringing us to the purpose of this guide. *This guide separates the facts from the fallacies about probiotics and natural human microecology.* In this way we hope to assist the reader in taking correct measures for improving, reaching, and maintaining optimal health.

# Antibiotics

## *State-of-the-Art Infection Fighters*

**ANTIBIOTIC** [from Greek *anti*, against + *bios*, life][1]

One of the greatest medical advances in the twentieth century is the discovery and use of antibiotics, which are considered to be the "drugs of choice" against bacterial and fungal infections. Indeed, the advent of antibiotics in the early 1940s initiated a new era of therapeutics for the treatment of human and animal microbial diseases. The microorganisms themselves generally produce these antibiotics for their sustenance in a given environmental niche. However, at present there are many antibiotics that are chemically synthesized.

Antibiotics can be codified into two major classes:

1. Narrow-spectrum antibiotics—useful against only a few classes of organisms
2. Broad-spectrum antibiotics—useful against a wide range of organisms

The use of antibiotics by health professionals has increased from 2 million pounds in the 1950s, to more than 50 million pounds today.[2] Antibiotics have turned many previously fatal bacterial diseases into treatable minor illnesses. Unfortunately, however, they have frequent side effects, and in recent times they have led to the development of antibiotic-resistant microorganisms. (See Figure 4 for benefits and side effects of a few commonly used antibiotics.) Robert S. Mendelson, M.D., summed this up in his book *Confessions of a Medical Heretic:* "By going too far . . . modern medicine has weakened and corrupted even the management of extreme cases. The miracle I and other doctors were once proud to take part in has become a miracle of mayhem."

Accordingly, in medical practice, the choice of any specific antibiotic is dependent not only on its effect on a particular infectious organism but also on consideration of the side, or toxic,

5

| PENICILLIN | AMOXYCILLIN | AMPICILLIN | KEFLEX |
|---|---|---|---|
| Antibiotic for a wide range of bacterial infections.<br><br>**Common side effects**: Sensitivity or allergic reaction.<br><br>**Less common side effects**: Upset stomach, nausea, vomiting, diarrhea, coating of the tongue, skin rash, itching, anemia, fungal diseases in mouth or rectum.<br><br>**Common penicillins used today**: Amoxicillin, ampicillin, bacampicillin, carbenicillin, cloxocillin, cyclacillin, dieloxacillin, hetacillin, methicillin, nafcillin, oxacillin, penicillin Gadoubee, penicillin V, ticarcillin | Antibiotic for bacterial infections such as pneumonia, venereal disease, meningitis; bloodstream, tonsil, and throat infections.<br><br>**Common side effects**: Upset stomach, nausea, vomiting, diarrhea, skin rash.<br><br>**Less common side effects**: Black "hairy" tongue, itching or irritation around anus and/or vagina and/or rectum. | Antibiotic for bacterial infections such as pneumonia, venereal disease, meningitis; tonsil and throat infections.<br><br>**Common side effects**: Upset stomach, nausea, vomiting, diarrhea, skin rash.<br><br>**Less common side effects**: "Hairy" tongue, itching or irritation around anus and/or vagina. | Antibiotic for infections of respiratory tract, middle ear, skin, bone, urinary tract.<br><br>**Common side effects**: Itching, rashes, fever, chills, blood reactions.<br><br>**Less common side effects**: Nausea, vomiting, diarrhea, abdominal cramps, upset stomach, headache, dizziness, difficulty breathing, tingling in the extremities, liver enlargement. |

| TETRACYCLINE | ERYTHROMYCIN | VIBRAMYCIN | NYSTATIN |
|---|---|---|---|
| Antibiotic for gonorrhea, bronchitis, pneumonia, urinary and other bacterial infections.<br><br>**Common side effects**: Upset stomach, nausea, vomiting, diarrhea, skin rash, "hairy" tongue, itching and irritation of anal and/or vaginal region.<br><br>**Less common side effects**: Loss of appetite, peeling of skin, sensitivity to sunlight, fever, chills, anemia, brown spotting of skin, liver damage, decrease in kidney function. | Antibiotic for respiratory tract, mouth, nose, ear, sinus, skin, and other bacterial infections.<br><br>**Common side effects**: Nusea, vomiting, stomach cramps, diarrhea, "hairy" tongue, itching, irritation of anal and/or vaginal region.<br><br>**Less common side effects**: Yellowing of skin and eyes. | Antibiotic for bacterial infections such as pneumonia, gonorrhea, bronchitis; fevers by ticks and lice; mouth and urinary tract infections.<br><br>**Common side effects**: Upset stomach, nausea, vomiting, diarrhea, skin rash, "hairy" tongue, itching and irritation of anal and/or vaginal region.<br><br>**Less common side effects**: Loss of appetite, peeling skin, sensitivity to the sun, fever, chills, anemia, brown spotting of skin, decrease in kidney function, liver damage. | Antifungal antibiotic against a wide variety of yeasts and yeastlike fungi.<br><br>**Occasionally produced side effects**: Diarrhea, gastrointestinal distresses, nausea, vomiting. |

**Figure 4: USES AND SIDE EFFECTS OF ANTIBIOTICS**[2, 3]

## CHLORAMPHENICOL

Antibiotic for infections susceptible to chloramphenicol. Prevents bacteria from growing or reproducing. Will not kill viruses.

*Life-threatening side effects*: Hives, rash, intense itching, fainting after a dose (anaphylaxis).

*Common side effects*: None expected.

*Less common side effects*: Pain, blurred vision, vision loss, swollen face or extremities; diarrhea; nausea; fever, jaundice, anemia, vomiting, numbness, tingling, burning pain or weakness in hands and feet, headache, confusion, sore throat.

## CIPROFLAXACIN

Antibiotic for infections of bone, gastrointestinal tract, lung, skin and soft tissue, urinary tract, gonorrhea.

*Life-threatening side effects*: Hives, rash, intense itching, fainting after a dose (anaphylaxis).

*Common side effects*: Abdominal discomfort, diarrhea, nausea, vomiting.

*Less common side effects*: Blurred vision, oral infections with yeast, unpleasant light-headedness, lower back pain, burning on urination, blood in urine, insomnia.

## NEOMYCIN

Antibiotic for clearing intestinal tract of germs prior to surgery; treats some causes of diarrhea, lowers blood cholesterol, lessens symptoms of hepatic coma.

*Common side effects*: Sore mouth, nausea, vomiting.

*Less common side effects*: Clumsiness, dizziness, rash, hearing loss, ringing or noises in ear, frothy stools, gaseousness, decreased frequency of urination.

## GRISEOFULVIN

Antibiotic for fungal infections.

*Common side effects*: Headaches.

*Less common side effects*: Confusion, rash, hives, itching, mouth or tongue irritation, soreness, nausea, vomiting, diarrhea, stomach pain, insomnia, tiredness, sore throat, fever, sensitivity to sunlight, numbness or tingling in hands and feet.

## CEPHALOSPORIN

Antibiotic for bacterial infections. Will not cure viral infections such as cold and flu.

*Life-threatening side effects*: Hives, rash, intense itching, fainting after a dose (anaphylaxis).

*Common side effects*: Difficult breathing, rash, redness, itching.

*Less common side effects*: Rectal itching, oral or vaginal candidiasis; mild nausea, vomiting, cramps; severe diarrhea with mucus or blood in stool; unusual weakness, tiredness; weight loss; fever.

## LINCOMYCIN

Antibiotic for bacterial infections.

*Common side effects*: None.

*Less common side effects*: Unusual thirst, vomiting, stomach cramps; severe and watery diarrhea with blood or mucus; painful swollen joints; jaundice, fever, tiredness, weakness, weight loss; rash; itch around groin, rectum, or armpits; white patches in mouth; vaginal discharge; itching.

## RIFAMYCIN

Antibiotic for tuberculosis and other infections. Requires daily use for 1 to 2 years.

*Common side effects*: Diarrhea; reddish urine, stool, saliva, sweat, and tears.

*Less common side effects*: Rash, flushed, itchy skin of face and scalp, blurred vision, difficult breathing, nausea, vomiting, abdominal cramps, dizziness, unsteady gait, confusion, muscle or bone pain, heartburn, flatulence, headache.

## STREPTOMYCIN

Originally developed to treat Gram-negative organisms resistant to penicillins. Was used in tuberculosis therapy.

*Side effects*: May produce toxic effects in liver or kidney. Allergic reactions frequent. Causes eighth nerve damage seen in vertigo and deafness; toxic reactions seen primarily in hearing and visual disturbances.

**USES AND SIDE EFFECTS OF ANTIBIOTICS (cont.)**

effects the antibiotic may cause, as well as the current condition of the patient's kidney function. Many antibiotics are given in lesser dosages or with greater intervals between dosages in the presence of impaired kidney function.

Another major concern about modern medicine's use of antibiotics is the development of antibiotic resistance by some pathogenic strains. According to Dr. Harold C. Neu of Columbia University in New York, "In 1941, a patient could receive 40,000 units of penicillin per day for 4 days and be cured of a case of Pneumococcal pneumonia. . . . Today, a patient could receive 24 million units of penicillin a day and die of Pneumococcal meningitis." He adds that bacteria that cause infection of the respiratory tract, skin, bladder, bowel, and blood . . . are now resistant to virtually all of the older antibiotics. The extensive use of antibiotics in the community and in hospitals has fueled this crisis."[3]

WHAT IS ANTIBIOTIC RESISTANCE?

Antibiotics kill the bacterial cells by attacking at different target sites. If there is any alteration within the bacteria, the antibiotic can no longer kill that organism and thus becomes resistant to that antibiotic.[4] This resistance to antibiotics has led to the proliferation of uncontrollable pathogenic microorganisms, reflected in greater mortality rates. Indeed, we are presently witnessing a massive, unprecedented, evolutionary change in bacteria.[5] We are in a new era of understanding; consideration of bacterial resistance must be part of our decision making and part of our planning for the future of antibiotic therapy.[6]

The misuse of antibiotics in health care is the main reason attributed to antibiotic resistance. For example, in the industrial world, though the antibiotics are available only by prescription, many people don't finish the course of treatment and conserve the leftovers to be used later.[7] Thus, next time they take the antibiotic, they take it in sublethal doses. These sublethal doses of antibiotics allow some of the bacteria to adapt in utilizing such sublethal concentrations of antibiotics as nutrients. Regular practice of ingesting such sublethal doses of antibiotics encourages the growth of the most resistant strains, which may later produce disorders that are very difficult to treat.

Some others have focused on the use of antibiotics among agricultural animals as the primary cause for this increased incidence of antibiotic resistance. For example, the same drugs prescribed for human therapy are widely used in animal husbandry. It has been estimated that, of the approximately 50 million pounds of antibiotics used, only one-half of that amount is used for human therapeutic purposes. The other half, or about 25 million pounds, are given to animals. This is either for treatment of various microbial infections or for the promotion of animal growth. As there are no specific guidelines for this use of antibiotics, excessive doses are frequently given to the animals, resulting in an accumulation of residual antibiotics in their bodies. Consequently, these antibiotics may enter the bloodstream of the animal and be secreted in meat and milk intended for human consumption.

In agriculture, antibiotics are applied also as aerosols to prevent bacterial infections. The lingering antibiotic residues can encourage the growth of resistant bacteria that later colonize in produce and are ingested by humans in their food.

Another concern is natural mutagenesis of organisms at the chromosomal level, which can lead to antibiotic resistance. Diverse sites within the bacterial cell serve as targets for the panoply of antibiotics used both clinically and in the agricultural community. In the antibiotic-resistant organism, contrary to its sensitive counterpart, an effective target is genetically changed, and this interrupts the drug-target interaction, leading to reduced effectiveness of the antibiotic on the organism.

Antibiotic resistance is not constrained by local or even national borders. It confronts all individuals and populations around the world. Misuse and overuse of antibiotics—whether in homes, hospitals, communities, in animal populations, or in agriculture—can provide the necessary environment to select and maintain resistant strains of bacteria. An approach to stem this tide is sorely needed.[7] The killing effect of antibiotics is so strong that only the resistant bacteria will survive.[8]

## Antibiotics and Attack of the Super Bugs
*by Bonnie C. Minsky*
September 2003

An antibiotic is a poison used to kill bacteria. Only licensed physicians can prescribe antibiotics. Unfortunately, antibiotics do not discriminate between unfriendly and friendly bacteria. Adult humans have about three to four pounds of friendly—or beneficial bacteria and yeast living in their intestinal tracts. If the beneficial bacteria are abundant, the unfriendly and pathogenic (disease-causing) ones remain in check. When in charge, beneficial bacteria fight harmful pathogens and produce B-vitamins.

When an oral antibiotic is swallowed, beneficial bacteria are killed, allowing yeast to grow unchecked in the intestines. Their tendrils poke holes in the lining of the intestinal walls creating a "leaky gut." Yeast can then escape and infiltrate other bodily tissues, causing suppression of the entire immune system.

Overuse and frequent misuse of antibiotics have created a serious situation of antibiotic resistance. Over prescribing by physicians is a major cause of antibiotic resistance. The U.S. Food and Drug Administration (FDA) estimates that half of the 100 million antibiotic prescriptions by U.S. physicians each year are unnecessary.

When prescribed for cold or flu, antibiotics are worthless; yet this is a common practice. According to several studies, children who were given antibiotics for acute ear infections suffered double the rate of adverse effects as compared to children who were given placebos. Antibiotics are also routinely prescribed for recurring sinus infections. Their benefit is merely transient, according to John Hopkins and Mayo Clinic researchers. They discovered that most recurring sinus infections are not caused by bacteria, but by fungi that are a type of yeast. Repeated use of antibiotics can encourage fungi to become deeply imbedded making them increasingly difficult to eradicate.

The FDA has become so alarmed about the overuse of antibiotic prescriptions, that antibiotic labels will soon bear a new warning that states the overuse of antibiotics will render them less effective. In addition, other health organizations, such as the Centers for Disease Control and the American Academy of Pediatrics, have published guidelines for physicians and consumers outlining the appropriate use of antibiotics.

A more hidden and insidious source of antibiotic resistance is the routine use of antibiotics in animal feed. More antibiotics are used for food animals—usually to encourage weight gain—than are used in all human medicine. Antibiotic resistance being transferred from food animals to humans is quite common. In addition, antibiotic residues found in many dairy products, eggs, meat, poultry, and farm-raised fish have caused resistant strains of salmonella, shigella, and other opportunistic pathogens.

In 2001, a scientific task force of microbiologists determined that "the presence of resistant bacteria in the GI tract are of particular concern because, not only do they act as a reservoir for antimicrobial resistance genes, but if established in other parts of the body, they can cause disease that cannot be treated." The problem could put a major strain on the entire healthcare system. Restricting farm practices that spread resistant genes is vital to curtailing this mounting health crisis.

We can all help physicians and governmental bodies to stop the overuse of antibiotics by taking these steps:

* Never take an antibiotic for a virus. Your doctor can order tests to definitively determine if an antibiotic is really necessary and which antibiotic, if needed, will prove the most successful.
* If an antibiotic is necessary, take the full course exactly as prescribed. Always take a probiotic, such as *Lactobacillus acidophilus*, after taking an antibiotic to restore beneficial bacteria.
* Avoid the long-term use of oral antibiotics for acne. There are many safer treatments available. Often, taking a natural anti-fungal preparation such as grapefruit seed extract or capryllic acid with probiotics and healthy dietary changes will arrest acne problems.
* Don't eat animal products from antibiotic treated animals. Certified organic animal foods are your safest choices. Even the fast food giant, McDonalds, has directed its meat suppliers to phase out the use of growth-promoting antibiotics in animals (although it doesn't serve organic products). (See *Choice News*, page 11, for more info on this.)
* Maintain a healthy immune system, which begins with eating a healthy diet.

The American public is drowning in an ocean of antibiotics. Remember that an ounce of prevention is worth a pound of cure, especially when the cure, in this case, actually encourages the attack of the super bugs.

*Bonnie Minsky is a Licensed and Certified Nutrition Specialist, Public Health Educator, and Certified Menopause Educator with a private practice in Northbrook, IL. She can be reached at nutritionalconcepts.com.*

© 2003–2004 CONSCIOUS CHOICE, 920 N. Franklin, Suite 202, Chicago, IL 60610, info@consciouschoice.com.

CAN WE REVERSE ANTIBIOTIC RESISTANCE?

There is strong evidence that antibiotics and antibacterials are used unnecessarily. Antimicrobial drugs, regardless of drug "category," should not be used for nontherapeutic purposes in food-producing animals. As multidrug resistance can emerge in as little as 7 days of chronic use of an antimicrobial drug, any rise in resistance levels that relates to antimicrobial drug use in food-producing animals could constitute a public health threat. Thus, the FDA must monitor resistance levels associated with animal-use antimicrobial drugs. According to Dr. S. B. Levy,[9] antibiotic resistance can be reduced to a great extent when consumers do not demand antibiotics, take them exactly as prescribed, and do not hoard them for later use. In addition, physicians should be judicious in prescribing antibiotics.

Another major way resistant strains may disappear is by competing with susceptible versions that persist in, or enter, a treated person after antibiotic use has stopped. In the absence of antibiotics, susceptible strains have a slight survival advantage because the resistant bacteria have to divert some of their valuable energy from reproduction to maintaining antibiotic-fighting traits. Ultimately, the susceptible microbes will win out, if they are available in the first place and are not killed off by more of the drug before they can prevail. Recommendations have been made to use probiotics or probiotic-producing microorganisms. Certain probiotics produce natural antibioticlike substances. Some researchers have termed these compounds *bacteriocins*, since they inhibit microbial growth. These compounds, mostly produced by lactic cultures, include Nisin produced by *Lactococcus lactis*, Diplococcin by *Lactococcus cremoris*, Acidophilin, Lactocidin, and Acidolin by *Lactobacillus acidophilus*, and Bulgarican from *L. bulgaricus*. Although little conclusive information is available concerning the detrimental effect of ingestion of such "natural" antibacterials, studies have suggested that the presence of such antibacterials in food products may be considered beneficial. They can increase the shelf life of foods, possibly inhibit the growth and toxin production of pathogenic organisms, and afford protection to the consumer against disease organisms. Additionally, the studies carried out in the author's laboratory, as well as by numerous other investigators, have established several nutritional and therapeutic aspects associated with such lactic acid bacteria. Thus, supplementation of useful bacteria in the form of probiotics can be a good prophylactic for chronic diseases caused by resistant pathogenic strains. The natural antibiotics produced by these probiotic cultures can eliminate any traces of resistant pathogens.

# Homeostasis

## A Balancing Act

**HOMEOSTASIS** [from Greek *homoios*, like, always the same, unchanging + *stasis*, standing]: *The maintenance of relatively stable internal physiological conditions (such as body temperature or the pH of the blood) in an organism, under fluctuating environmental conditions. Homeostasis is achieved by a system of control mechanisms within the organism.*[1, 2]

The human organism constantly strives to maintain homeostasis—its natural balance. It has the ability to resist almost all types of organisms or toxins that tend to damage cells, tissues, and organs. This capacity is called immunity.[3]

At birth, the human intestinal tract of the newborn is described as "sterile"—devoid of microbes. However, beginning with its passage through the birth canal, it progressively becomes inhabited with microbes of various species, depending on the type of food ingested. These microbes are derived first from the mother during breast-feeding and later from many other outside sources.

During breast-feeding, the beneficial bifidobacteria and Gram-positive lactobacilli begin to appear. The mother is "jump-starting" the baby's immunity. Breasts have colostrum in them when a mother is pregnant, and that is what the baby gets when he first sucks, until the mother's milk comes in. The colostrum carries antibodies from the mother's blood, so temporary immunities are passed on to the baby. It also has protein, sugar, fat, vitamins, and minerals in it. Colostrum is yellowish and turns to white milk around the second or third day after birth.

After the baby is born, the mother's pituitary gland produces a hormone called prolactin. This hormone induces the milk to come in a few days after birth. The baby's nuzzling, licking, and sucking on the nipples tends to stimulate the release of another pituitary hormone, oxytocin, which prompts the "let-down reflex," causing the milk to flow or squirt. The breast milk works on a supply/demand basis: The more the baby sucks, the more milk will be made.[4]

It is universally agreed that when the human organism is healthy (in its state of natural homeostatic balance) its breast milk cannot be surpassed as food for babies.[5] Breast milk is the best possible nutrition for all babies—full term, premature, healthy, or ill. It is more than just a standard. It is the only truly compatible, truly nutritious food a newborn can eat.[6] Breast milk is perfectly suited to the baby's needs and digestion—it is almost germ-free when produced, it goes directly to the consumer without being handled, and it is always fresh. Breast milk contains protective antibodies, antiviral properties, and vitamins. Lactoferrin in breast milk has a bacteriostatic effect on *E. coli*. Breast-fed babies have fewer illnesses during the first year of life. Breast-feeding reduces the risk of hypocalcemia and milk allergy.[7] When there is natural balance in the mother, there are qualitative and quantitative differences in the intestinal flora of infants who are exclusively breast fed and those who are bottle fed. Exclusively breast-fed infants experience markedly fewer gastrointestinal upsets or diarrheal incidents than formula-fed infants. It is well known that bifidobacterium is the predominant microbe in the intestinal tract of breast-fed infants; it is responsible for their reduced diarrhea frequencies.[8] During weaning, the flora undergo a permanent change to a more diversified flora made up of bacteroides, clostridium, escherichia, lactobacilli, and streptococci.[9] The resulting disturbances in bowel microecology are one cause of diarrhea.

The situation today is often quite different from the natural homeostatic scenario described in the paragraphs above. Today, even as early as at the time of birth, the natural balance has often already been disrupted in the mother; therefore, it is disrupted in the infant.

German research shows that the state of the intestinal flora in most breast-fed babies today is similar to that of formula-fed babies 40 years ago. The result is malabsorption and food sensitivity problems as well as an increase in allergies and susceptibility to infection. Further research has pointed to contamination of breast milk with pollutants such as DDT, dioxin[10], as well as numerous other chemical toxins. This suggests that probiotic supplementation for all babies may now be an appropriate strategy.

At birth and throughout life, the large intestine is a bacterium's idea of paradise. The human gut provides food, shelter, and warmth for these microbes to proliferate.

Most of us are aware of the changes that have occurred in the outer world of Earth today—the macroecology. Just as toxic chemicals have harmed the macroecology, for many of us, our inner world—the microecology of the gastrointestinal system—has also been harmed and changed.

As well as being one of the most commonly prescribed classes of drugs, one-half of the antibiotics produced in America today end up in the meat we eat.[11] Beyond the serious situation cited earlier (where antibiotic overuse leads to the development of resistant bacterial strains), antibiotics disrupt our natural microecological balance in another serious way.

Unfortunately, "good" flora are quite vulnerable to antibiotics, and are often killed along with the "bad" flora that are targeted by antibiotic therapy. When this happens, numerous other health complications can occur.

The situation is similar to what happens when we interfere with nature's "ecological balance" in the outer world. Man destroys too many of a certain species of an animal, for instance. An insect that this animal normally eats can then become over-populous, causing some harm. Allowing the animals to again increase to normal numbers eliminates the problem with the insects, and balance is restored.[12]

In the human system, one of the most common microbial forms to overpopulate is a yeast called *Candida albicans*. Another is an organism called *Clostridium botulinum* (the source of toxins that cause botulism). Others include those which cause Salmonella and Shigella diarrheas.

These opportunistic organisms, once they gain a foothold and start growing, can cause a wide range of health problems. Besides antibiotics, poor nutrition that leads to imbalances, deficiencies, and toxicities can also impair immunity or resistance and result in overcolonization of these undesirable floras. In other words, by destroying or interfering with the "good guys" that keep the undesirables "under control," the undesirables instead become too prolific.[13]

Therefore, the flora problem has three aspects to it:

1. Undercolonization and destruction of the desirable flora — the probiotics.
2. Overcolonization and development of the undesirable flora.
3. Development of new undesirable and resistant strains.

A vicious cycle of dysbiosis, or microflora imbalance, is then set up in the internal microbiological terrain of the GI system.

It now becomes clear when researching the question "What constitutes health?" that an adequate balance and population of bacteria that normally inhabit the gastrointestinal tract are fundamental components of the answer.

An imbalance sets the stage for a cascade of events that may lead to the onset and progression of many disease conditions. Therefore, it is essential to human health that a probiotic gastrointestinal environment be established and maintained.

# Introducing the Probiotics

## *Friendly Flora: What Are They?*

**PROBIOTIC** [from Greek *pro*, supporting + *bios*, life][1, 2]

Establishing a probiotic gastrointestinal environment refers to maintaining those microorganisms in our gut that prevent or reduce the effects of an infection caused by pathogenic organisms.[3] These "friendly flora" also help us digest the food we eat. The bad bacteria are the ones that are just trying to survive, and in doing so they produce their own toxins.

To be effective, a probiotic must increase/multiply itself in the host's gut, while decreasing/destroying the number and the effect of the disease-producing organisms already present in the gut.

The word "probiotic" means "for life," but in the context of intestinal health, probiotics often refer to the dietary supplements of friendly bacteria that can be taken in pill or powder form to enhance and support good intestinal functioning. These supplements of friendly bacteria are actually supplements of life forms. Like other life forms, they consume and utilize resources; they produce and excrete wastes; they reproduce themselves; and eventually they die.

The good bacteria are known as probiotic for a reason: They help support life. They have a job to perform, and without them life would be impossible. (See Figure 5 for some friendly bacteria.)

The many varieties of bacteria that are essential to intestinal health are broadly called "lactic acid" or "lactic bacteria" (LAB). Lactic bacteria have the ability to transform sugar into lactic acid. Lactic acid is one of the antibioticlike substances used by the lactic bacteria to kill off other undesirable bacteria.

There are many species that belong to the group of lactic acid bacteria. These include *L. acidophilus, L. bulgaricus, L. salivarius,*

| LACTOBACILLUS ACIDOPHILUS | LACTOBACILLUS BULGARICUS | LACTOBACILLUS PLANTARUM | OTHER COMMONLY USED LACTOBACILLUS PROBIOTICS |
|---|---|---|---|
| Initiates the implantation and colonization of bacteria, primarily in the colon. Known to be able to produce natural antibiotics, including antiviral compounds. Controls pH in the colon. The patented special strain DDS-1 is unique and superior to other strains of acidophilus. DDS-1 is resistant to heat and the extreme conditions in the intestines.<br><br>*Common side effects*: None known. | *L. bulgaricus* is usually used in combination with *Streptococcus thermophilus* to ferment natural yogurt, which has been proven beneficial in promoting health and increasing longevity.<br><br>*Common side effects*: None known. | An important part of the "good guy" bacteria constantly waging warfare with "bad" bacteria in the intestines. Assists *L. acidophilus* in combating pathogens. Has unique ability to synthesize L-lysine, an amino acid known for beneficial attributes.<br><br>*Common side effects*: None known. | *Lactobacillus rueteri*: It is more powerful than *L. acidophilus* as a natural antibiotic.<br><br>*Lactobacillus salivarius*: Salivarius has been shown to help in the majority of chronic conditions related to the bowel and in strengthening the immune system.<br><br>*Lactobacillus brevis*<br><br>*Common side effects*: None known. |

| BIFIDOBACTERIUM | OTHER COMMONLY USED BIFIDOBACTERIUM | ENTEROCOCCUS FAECIUM | STREPTOCOCCCUS THERMOPHILUS |
|---|---|---|---|
| Extensive research documents its benefits. *Bifidobacterium bifidum* is a powerful bacteria that assists in the detoxification and suppression of pathogens.<br><br>*Common side effects*: None known. | *Bifidobacterium infantis*<br><br>*Bifidobacterium longus*<br><br>*Bifidobacterium breve*<br><br>*Common side effects*: None known. | The most durable of these microorganisms. It has such a strong stabilization, it is able to resist the high acidic levels and temperatures in the stomach. Research shows that even under the most extreme conditions some implantation of this beneficial bacteria is achieved. Not only that, it supports the other bacteria, helping them to survive and be implanted as well.<br><br>*Common side effects*: None known. | Usually used along with *L. bulgaricus* to manufacture yogurt. *S. thermophilus* bacteria produces abundant amounts of the enzyme lactase and is very effective in preventing lactose intolerance. |

**Figure 5: KNOWN BENEFICIAL BACTERIA**[4, 5, 6]

## HELPFUL OR DESIRABLE BACTERIA
## (PROBIOTICS), INCLUDING LAB

Includes Lactic-Acid-Producing Bacteria (LAB):

### *Bifidobacterium (B.)*
- *B. bifidum*
- *B. infantis*
- *B. longum*
- *B. breve*

### *Lactobacillus (L.)*
- *L. acidophilus*
- *L. plantarum*
- *L. salivarius*
- *L. bulgaricus*
- *L. brevis*
- *L. casei*
- *L. rhamnosus*

### *Streptococcus (S.)*
- *S. thermophilus*

### *Enterococcus (E.)*
- *E. faecium*

---

### UNDESIRABLE BACTERIA (Potential Pathogens)

Clostridium

Escherichia (some strains)

Coliform

Staphylococcus

Pseudomonas

---

### NONPATHOGENIC—NONCOMMITTAL (Neither good nor bad)

Bacteriodes

---

### Figure 6: COMMON INTESTINAL FLORA AND SPECIFIC SPECIES

and others. Each species has hundreds of strains; the DDS-1 strain of *L. acidophilus* has been studied extensively by the author, Dr. Khem Shahani.

Of all the friendly bacteria that help the human body, most are residents, while others are transient visitors, staying in the digestive tract for a few weeks before passing on.

In the adult there are six major groups of bacteria that inhabit the gastrointestinal tract. Those that produce lactic acid tend to promote health. The others tend to cause disease when lactic acid bacteria are in short supply (see Figure 6).

While nearly twenty or more species of the so-called "friendly" bacteria have been identified, only the most commonly occurring ones have undergone scientific evaluation. To date, these principal forms of scientifically validated friendly bacteria are the following:

### (1) Lactobacillus acidophilus

[From the Latin *lactis*, milk; *bacillus*, little rod; *acidum*, acid; from the Greek *philein*, to love.] This is the primary bacteria in the "friendly" class, and is the main inhabitant of the lower small intestinal area in humans and animals. It is also found in the mouth and vagina. Its significant health-giving properties will be explained in detail later.

The lactobacilli constitute one of the six major groups of intestinal and fecal microorganisms in humans as well as animals. Under favorable and healthy conditions there are more than 100 billion of these health-promoting bacteria thriving in the gut.[7]

### (2) Lactobacillus plantarum

*L. plantarum* is a *transient*, or nonresident, bacteria found in humans. It is also found in dairy products and pickled vegetables. It is an important part of the "good guy" bacteria that constantly engage in warfare with "bad" bacteria in the intestines. It has the distinctive feature of synthesizing L-lysine. It produces lactic acid, creating a poor environment for "bad" bacteria.

### (3) Lactobacillus salivarius

*L. salivarius* is found in humans and chickens. It has been shown to help in almost all chronic conditions related to the bowel, primarily by creating an acidic environment.

### (4) Lactobacillus bulgaricus

Many cultures throughout the world that utilize large quantities of this bacteria have reported increased longevity, greater health, prolonged functioning of the internal organs, as well as other benefits. It is known to cooperate with *L. acidophilus* to establish a protective colonization of the intestinal tract.

This is a transient but very important bacteria. Together with *Streptococcus thermophilus*, it is used to make yogurt.

### (5) Lactobacillus rueteri

Very similar to *L. acidophilus*, it has the greatest ability to react and survive in various conditions. It is also likely to be the most potent antibiotic that is able to deal with organisms. *L. rueteri* is a specialty organism whose benefits have been researched by Dr. Speck at North Carolina State University—one of the top probiotic authorities in the world.

### (6) Lactobacillus brevis

*L. brevis* is a transient bacteria of the human intestines. It is naturally found in milk, cheese, and cow intestines. It produces a strongly acidic environment.

### (7) Bifidobacterium bifidum, infantis, breve, and longum

[From the Latin *bifid*, into two parts or branches; *infans*, infant; *brevis*, short; *longus*, long.] Bifidobacteria are the main inhabitants of the large intestine. *B. bifidum* is also found in the vagina and lower part of the small intestine. In breast-fed infants and adolescents these bifidobacteria make up 99 percent of the entire flora of the bowel; whereas lactobacilli, enterococci, and coliforms comprise about 1 percent (actually these can range from 1–15%) of the large intestine's flora.

Bifidobacteria are a major component of the large intestinal flora from adolescence through adulthood, but are usually outnumbered by bacteroides. Lactobacilli, enterococci, and coliforms are a smaller component of the flora in this bowel area.

Although lactobacilli are found in smaller numbers than bifidobacteria in the intestines, they carry out important metabolic activities. They are particularly important in the small intestine where they are a normal resident. Bifidobacteria are reduced significantly in the stools of old people, but clostridia, streptococci, and coliforms increase.[8]

There is strong evidence that the numbers and efficient working of these bacteria decline as a person ages and with any decline in our health status.

### (8) *Streptococcus thermophilus*

[From the Greek *streptos*, twisted; Latin *cocci*, round.] A transient bacteria of the human intestines, it is naturally found in dairy products, and together with *L. bulgaricus* it produces yogurt. Because it produces large amounts of lactase and is very efficient in breaking down lactose, consumption of *S. thermophilus* is particularly helpful to lactose-intolerant people.

### (9) *Enterococcus faecium*

[From the Greek *entero*, intestine; Latin *cocci*, round.] *E. faecium* is a transient bacteria in the human intestine. It is naturally found in animals and plants, and is used as a starter culture for some cheeses. The most durable of the organisms discussed here because it has the ability to adapt to a variety of conditions and still survive, it tolerates a wide range of pH and temperature, and is very stable over extreme conditions. Reliable research and literature show that, even under the worst conditions, some implementation of this beneficial bacteria is achieved.

## Gut Bacteria, the Immune System, and Sleep

"Your immune system and bacteria, in the same twenty-four-hour period, have the same need for tension and resolution [as does your feast-or-famine metabolism]."

- Two-and-a-half to four pounds of bacteria inhabit our gut at any given time.
- We evolved symbiotically with this microflora as a primary expression of our immune system.
- Our "personal bacteria" are constantly at war with pathogenic bacteria and viruses.
- The battle in our gut is waged mostly at night when high levels of by-products of the bacteria trigger our immune systems to reduce the levels of bacteria, particularly the harmful species.
- During the daylight hours, the bacteria feed and multiply on carbohydrate sugars; sunlight, expressed as energy cells delivered to the gut; and reproductive hormones.
- Sleep is triggered through the same immune system reaction that "thins the herd" of our gut bacteria
- Darkness and closed eyes during sleep stimulate melatonin production, which encourages white blood cell activity designed to respond to pathogens like the harmful bacteria in your gut.
- Prolactin synthesis, in deep sleep, further contributes to immune system mobilization.
- When you are ill and your gut microflora is out of balance, you sleep more to increase the production of white blood cells, "T" cells, and Natural Killer cells.

Conclusions:

- The gut microflora are influenced directly by circadian rhythms of the environment and the body. This rhythm is an essential part of a healthy immune system.
- To be healthy and have a balanced internal ecology, we need to get plenty of sunshine during the day and sleep at night.

Source: *Lights Out!* T. S. Wiley and Bent Formby, Ph.D., NY: Pocket Books, 2000, pp. 48–51, 53.

# Probiotics and Human Nutrition

## *A Long Tradition*

For centuries, lactic acid bacteria have been used in the preservation of food for human consumption. Indeed, historically, fermented milk products have constituted a vital component of the human diet for many throughout Asia, Eastern Europe, and Africa. The main objective of fermenting milk has been to preserve this precious fluid which otherwise would deteriorate rapidly under the high temperatures of the Middle East, where this process is likely to have originated.

Yogurt, which results from the fermentation of milk by lactic acid bacteria, is one of the oldest and most popular cultured dairy products worldwide. Yogurt is a semisolid product made from milk by the activity of a symbiotic blend of *Streptococcus thermophilus* and *Lactobacillus delbruecki* [subspecies *bulgaricus* (LB)] cultures. Basic yogurt is nothing more than milk to which a dose of harmless bacteria has been added. The bacteria produce an enzyme called lactase. This enzyme attacks or hydrolyzes the natural milk sugar, lactose—the first step on the way to production of lactic acid. The acid then lowers the pH and gently curdles the milk as it imparts a tart flavor.[1] The milk of various mammals is used for making yogurt; however, most of the industrial production of yogurt uses cow's milk.

In many parts of the world yogurt is still made at home from traditional kitchen recipes involving milk from cows, water buffaloes, goats, sheep, mare, or camel. The milk is boiled, cooled, and inoculated with yogurt left over from the previous day, and incubated at ambient temperature for 4 to 6 hours, until it acquires a thick consistency. It is then utilized for consumption in the fresh state as a snack, as an accompaniment, as a salad containing fresh vegetables (carrots, cucumber, etc.), as a sweet or savory drink, or as a dessert containing seasonal fruits.

Only recently has this cultured dairy food gained favor in the United States. Yogurt has now emerged as a significant dairy product. In the past two decades we have witnessed a dramatic increase in annual yogurt consumption, from nearly 1 pound to 4.2 pounds per capita.

These foods, like yogurt fermented with bacteria (especially those with lactobacilli), are of great importance as they are a source of dietary probiotics.

Anecdotal health claims from regular consumption of cultured dairy products circulated for centuries without scientific proof. Then in 1908, Russian Professor Elie Metchnikoff, a Nobel prize recipient who discovered phagocytes (the white blood cells that defend in our immune system), provided scientific evidence that the probiotic microorganisms may be responsible for these health claims.

Metchnikoff studied the history of yogurt, finding that it dated back to the dawn of civilization. Bulgarians, Serbs, and others had made it not only from cow's milk but also from sheep, goat, and buffalo milk; Russians had made it from mare's milk; and the Finns and others made it from reindeer and yak milk.

Metchnikoff was enchanted by the fact that so many people in Bulgarian villages lived beyond 100 years, and he wanted to know why. This longevity of the Bulgarians, he found, could be attributed to their regular consumption of large quantities of yogurt fermented with lactic-acid-producing bacteria, which inhibit pathogens and detoxify their systems. He appropriately named these bacteria "*L. bulgaricus.*"

He similarly credited the exceptional longevity of the Balkan people to this organism. Several years passed before studies were done to determine the details of why all this was so.[2] It is fortuitous that what Metchnikoff theorized at the beginning of the century (1908), Shahani and his associates established at the end of the century. Indeed, lactobacilli contribute to the longevity of life.

Today there is a steady flow of scientific findings supporting this conclusion.

# The Role of Probiotics in Human Nutrition

As stated earlier, food is normally digested partially in the mouth, stomach, and finally in the intestine, where the partially digested food is ultimately metabolized (broken down) by billions of microorganisms (the probiotics) working simultaneously, synergistically, and symbiotically with other agents.

Under favorable, healthy conditions the probiotics are present in large numbers, but in an unhealthy or diseased situation, the pathogenic organisms dominate.

The friendly bacteria do not just take up residence in the gut and do nothing in return. They live in symbiosis with our bodies, performing many important functions in the body. As long as we provide the bacteria with a healthy food supply, and as long as they stay healthy, these bacteria perform important services in return.

Numerous research studies have revealed various specific nutritional and therapeutic properties attributable to the probiotic organisms. The recognition and clarification of these properties has revealed that there does exist variation in benefits among different species—and even wide variation among different strains of the same species.

While working with probiotics over the past 40 years, we have been able to substantiate and categorize the actual probiotics with their beneficial properties.

SPECIFIC NUTRITIONAL AND THERAPEUTIC PROPERTIES OF
PROBIOTICS: WHAT THEY DO AND HOW THEY WORK

## (1) Alleviate Anxiety

The presence of lactic-acid-producing organisms may also explain a report that cultured dairy products help relieve anxiety. This benefit may be due not only to the steady biosynthesis of B vitamins, but also to the high production of the amino acid tryptophan during fermentation. Tryptophan is known to relieve anxiety through synthesis of the neurotransmitter serotonin.[3]

## (2) Assist Digestion of the Major Food Components—Fats, Carbohydrates, and Proteins

Among the many health benefits of ingesting lactic acid bacteria is the nutritional bioavailability enhancements to which they contribute. Nutritional bioavailability refers to the availability, absorption, retention, and utilization of nutrients to the human organism's benefit.[4]

The probiotic organisms actually help us utilize our food. Having their own inherent capacity to multiply/propagate, they naturally digest food. They can't *directly* digest food for us, but because they want to grow and flourish, they are actually utilizing the food available in our GI systems for themselves; in doing so, they leave the predigested food to provide energy for us.

In order to do all this digesting, they produce their own enzymes. They even leave enzymes behind for us to use; we use them to further break down food particles.[5]

In this capacity, probiotics improve:

- *The digestion and absorption of fat by the production of lipases*—lipases are the primary fat-digesting enzymes.

- *The digestion of carbohydrates, especially the lactose in milk.* Approximately 30 percent of lactose in milk is hydrolyzed by lactase from lactic acid bacteria. This is one of the reasons for increased tolerance, by lactose-intolerant individuals, of fermented dairy products.[6]

- *Protein tolerance.* Lactobacilli have been shown to hydrolyze protein, creating significantly higher levels of free essential amino acids as compared to unfermented milk.[7] Protein intolerance is a commonly reported complaint when intestinal bacteria are out of balance. Toxins that decrease the number of viable, health-promoting bacteria also interfere with digestive enzymes. Complex proteins are especially difficult to digest under these compromised conditions, which may largely account for allergies to milk and eggs, and the widespread occurrence of celiac disease (an allergic reaction to the complex protein gluten found in rye, barley, oats, and wheat). The preferred sources of protein then, for sufferers of protein intolerance, are rice and soybeans (which are free of gluten), flours made only from these grains, and foods that contain predigested, free amino acids (such as yogurt, cultured dairy products, and eggs) which are easier to digest than complete, complex proteins.[8]

- *Production of the enzyme lactase, which increases lactose tolerance.* Of all the food sensitivities, one of the most common is lactose intolerance. In fact, up to 70 percent of the world's population may develop gastrointestinal symptoms following the consumption of lactose-containing dairy foods.[9] Such reactions occur because these people have a deficiency of the enzyme lactase, which is necessary to digest lactose. Lactase is an enzyme secreted normally in the small intestine, but its production shows a steady decline with age after weaning.[10] People who suffer from lactose intolerance malabsorb milk lactose in the small intestine, so lactose is passed on to the large intestine where lactic-acid-forming bacteria digest it.

However, even here the success of digesting lactose requires that intestinal bacteria are healthy and present in sufficient quantity. When the large intestine is deficient in health-promoting bacteria, the undigested lactose overwhelms the ability to digest it, causing an increase in osmotic pressure. Also, the undigested lactose is metabolized by colonic bacteria to yield hydrogen, methane, and other gases. This is believed to account for the pain, diarrhea, gas, and related gastrointestinal symptoms that characterize lactose intolerance.

Cultured dairy products are tolerated better than whole milk because they contain less lactose (due to predigestion by lactase) and because of the presence of lactase-producing microorganisms.

### (3) Produce Natural Antibioticlike Agents; Fight and Prevent Miscellaneous Bacterial Infections

Lactic acid and other products secreted by lactic-acid-forming bacteria tend to suppress the growth of pathogenic bacteria while having little effect on healthful bacteria.

When the human intestinal system gets out of balance, the unfriendly bacteria produce toxic substances that have detrimental effects on the overall system's health and function.

*In vitro* studies have indicated that lactic acid bacteria favorably alter the gastrointestinal microecology.[11] The change in intestinal microecology may in part be due to antimicrobial substances produced by LAB and/or their continuous consumption. The inhibition of pathogens *in vitro* is due to lactic acid, hydrogen peroxide, and/or antimicrobial substances produced by lactic acid bacteria.[12]

Bifidobacteria produce acetic and lactic acids as metabolites. The production of these acids reduces intestinal pH, which in turn restricts or prohibits the growth of many potentially pathogenic and putrefactive bacteria. Bifidobacteria induce more antimicrobial activity than lactobacilli because they produce more acetic acid (3:2 acetic to lactic), a higher amount of which exists in undissaociated (usable) form at the intestinal pH, thereby exerting higher antimicrobial activity.[13]

*L. bulgaricus* produces the natural antibiotic bulgarican, which initiates antibacterial activity against several Gram-positive and Gram-negative organisms, including pathogens; however, it has no apparent antifungal activity.

*L. acidophilus* produces lactic acid, which suppresses undesirable bacteria and yeasts. Some strains produce the natural antibioticlike agent, acidophilin. This natural substance is active against a wide variety of Gram-positive and Gram-negative pathogenic organisms.

Polonskaya[14] observed that *L. acidophilus* has the capacity to inhibit the growth of common disease-causing organisms such as *Salmonella, Shigella, Enterococcus faecalis,* and *E. coli.* In addition to acidophilin, some strains of *L. acidophilus* secrete other natural antibiotics: acidolin, lactocidin and bacterlocin.

*L. plantarum* secretes lactolin. *L. brevis* secretes lactobacillin and lactobrevin.

Additionally, the bacteriocidal property of lactobacilli can partially be credited to the initiation of the lactoperoxidase system. Lactoperoxidase acts on thiocyanate to produce $H_2O_2$ (hydrogen peroxide), which in turn kills bacteria. Similarly, a thiosulfinate component of the oil of garlic, known as Allicin, has proven to have bactericidal and antifungal properties.[15] Therefore, if garlic and lactobacilli of the right species and strain are present in sufficient quantity and combination, the invading pathogen is killed. This largely explains the effective synergism of garlic and the intestinal bacteria that exists in killing waterborne and foodborne pathogens.

The probiotics are effective against both Gram-positive and Gram-negative microorganisms. Inhibition of the growth of 27 toxin-producing microorganisms has been proven.[16] These pathogenic microorganisms are members of the following genera: Sarcina, Serratia, Proteus, Coliform, Shigella, Pseudomonas, Staphylococcus, Klebsiella, and Vibrio.[17]

In treating 19 cases of nonspecific infection of the vagina with acidophilus, 95 percent were cured. In 25 cases of monila vaginitis, 88 percent were cured and 12 percent were relieved of symptoms. In 444 cases of trichomonas vaginitis, 92 percent were cured and remained infection-free up to a year later.[18]

The antibioticlike substance, acidophilin, which *L. acidophilus* naturally produces, will kill 50 percent of 27 different disease-causing bacteria.[19]

*Enterococcus faecium*, which has also been shown to be a very good probiotic that produces antimicrobial substances, relieves diarrhea, augments immune responses, and provides synergistic and supplementary/complimentary effects with *Lactobacillus acidophilus*.[20] This particular culture has been used very effectively at the International Center for Diarrhea Disease Research in Bangladesh (ICDDRB).[21]

*L. acidophilus* grows in the vagina in large numbers and maintains an acidic pH there.[22] The vaginal microflora change drastically during bacterial infection.[23] Bacteria of the genera Escherichia, Proteus, Klebsiella, and Pseudomonas, along with yeast, *Candida albicans*, are recognized as etiological agents in urinary tract infections among adult women. Guillot[24] speculated that *L. acidophilus* could produce metabolites that retard the growth of *C. albicans.* Collins and Hardt[25] suggested that *L. acidophilus* suppressed the growth of *C. albicans* through production of antimicrobial substances.

Considerable progress has been made in understanding the urinary tract infection mechanism and the ability of *Lactobacillus* sp. to circumvent the diseased state. Wood et al.[26] showed that various species of lactobacilli were able to adhere *in vitro* to vaginal epithelial cells—with no difference among strains detected. The uropathogens adhere to the epithelium before the onset of the disease.[27]

Adherence is governed by host and bacterial cell properties.[28, 29] Shand et al.[30] provided the *in vivo* evidence that iron-restricted conditions are important regarding the growth of bacteria involved in urinary tract infection. Chan et al.[31] have shown that the normal urethral, vaginal, and cervical flora of healthy females can competitively block the attachment of uropathogenic bacteria to the surfaces of uroepithelial cells in women with and without a history of urinary tract infection. The lactobacilli that coat the uroepithelium prevent the uropathogen attachments to their receptors. This suggests that the normal flora of the urinary tract may be used to protect against the attachment of uropathogens to the surface of uroepithelial cells.

### (4) Prevent Arterial Disease, Lower Cholesterol, and Improve HDL/LDL Ratio

Cholesterol is found in every cell membrane of all animals, and it plays an important role in the normal metabolic process of man. It is essential for the biosynthesis of several steroid hormones, such as sex and adrenal hormones, as well as bile acids. The body produces cholesterol in larger amounts than that contributed by dietary sources. Cholesterol is synthesized in accordance with the body's requirement for it.

A high serum cholesterol level is linked to increased consumption of dairy and animal fats and to a significant increase in the number of deaths from atherosclerotic heart disease.[32] Half of all deaths in the United States are caused by atherosclerosis, the disease in which cholesterol accumulates in the walls of arteries, forming bulky plaques that inhibit the flow of blood until a clot eventually forms, obstructing an artery and causing a heart attack. The cholesterol of atherosclerosis plaques is derived from particles called low-density lipoproteins (LDL) that circulate in the bloodstream. The more LDL there is in the blood, the more rapid atherosclerosis develops.[33] Conversely, high-density lipoprotein (HDL) is associated with low rates of coronary heart disase.[34] Suggestions have been made that HDL plays an important role in the removal of tissue cholesterol.[35]

Hypercholesteremia is considered to be one of the major factors predisposing an individual to atherosclerotic heart disease, and it has also been widely accepted that diet can play a significant role in reducing cholesterol.

Studies in our laboratory have indicated that the ingestion of fermented milk and acidophilus resulted in the reduction of serum cholesterol. A graduate student in the author's group found, while studying hypercholesterolemic individuals, that fermented milk caused a distinct increase in the HDL/LDL ratio[36]—a change that is beneficial to heart health, but seldom obtained by following the usual low-fat, low-cholesterol diet.

Researchers who studied the Masai tribes of Kenya discovered a possible mode of action for this. While the Masai eat an abundance of animal products and consume large quantities of fermented milk, their average total cholesterol level and incidence of heart disease is much lower than that of people in Western countries.

Ahmed et al.[37] credited the cholesterol-lowering effect of fermented milk to orotic acid, which is present in whey, and has since been shown to serve as an inhibitor of hepatic biosynthesis of cholesterol. Yet as Grunewald was to demonstrate, the cholesterol-lowering effect of these organisms is highly subject to strain specificity.[38] Therefore, the strain of lactobacilli used to make yogurt may or may not have the same beneficial effect as that used by the Masai tribes.

Tortuero et al.[39] found that feeding *L. acidophilus* to laying hens resulted in a significant decrease in serum cholesterol. Harrison and Peet[40] observed a similar effect when they fed a milk formula supplemented with *L. acidophilus* to infants. In another study, the addition of 4 million *L. acidophilus* DDS-1 cells per milliliter of milk lowered cholesterol significantly.[41]

Based on the evidence cited here, it seems wise to include cultured dairy foods and supplements rich in viable lactobacilli in any cholesterol-lowering regimen.

### (5) Fight Childhood and Adult Dysentery

Fermented dairy products containing viable lactobacilli have been used by humans primarily as a prophylactic aid, and their use has been extended to intestinal infections. About 40–70 percent of the children with Salmonella and Shigella dysentery recovered when acidophilus milk was administered for a short period of time. Continued long-term administration of acidophilus milk resulted in 100 percent recovery.[42]

Alm[43] observed that the oral administration of *L. acidophilus* reduced the carrier time (time during which a person carries the bacteria but shows no symptoms) in children and in adults infected with Salmonella.

Several researchers have suggested that fermented dairy products and viable lactobacilli may be more efficacious in treating gastrointestinal disorders than the administration of antibiotics.[44, 45, 46]

### (6) Fight Infant Dysentery

Dietary lactobacilli also have been used for the treatment of infantile diarrhea.[47]

### (7) Inhibit Food Pathogens and Enhance Food Preservation

*In vitro*, there is a scientific consensus that LAB (lactic acid bacteria) are antagonistic toward foodborne pathogens. The foodborne pathogens produce toxins in food, resulting in food intoxication, or they may multiply in food to cause infection. LAB may hinder the proliferation of some foodborne pathogens in the food system.[48]

Following colonization by pathogenic bacteria, the numbers of undesired bacteria increase and the numbers of beneficial bacteria, such as lactobacilli and streptococci, decrease. Ingestion of *L. acidophilus* and *Enterococcus faecium* supplements other sources of viable lactobacilli and favorably alters the gut microecology. Lactic-acid-producing bacteria also produce antimicrobial substances that inhibit the growth of invasive pathogenic bacteria.[49] Therefore, establishment of LAB in the gastrointestinal tract may provide prophylactic and therapeutic benefits against intestinal infections. Prophylaxis may have some beneficial role in circumventing traveler's diarrhea.

One cause of gastrointestinal disturbance is the alteration in the intestinal microbiota following invasion or infection by foodborne pathogens. The decrease in the coliform count has been attributed to the low pH produced by the lactic acid present in yogurt and acidified milk base.[50] Some pathogens must establish and/or colonize the gastrointestinal tract before the onset of the disease. LAB may hinder the colonization and subsequent proliferation of the foodborne pathogens, thereby preventing the disease state. Traditionally, this rationale has been used for treating diseases with fermented milk products (FMP). Further, FMP reduce the number or eliminate the foodborne pathogens that potentially may produce toxins in the food system and the gastrointestinal tract by elaborating antimicrobial substances. The production of antimicrobial substances is dependent on the genera, species, strain, incubation medium, and other conditions.[51]

Bifidobacteria and acidophilus kill most food-poisoning bacteria, so these can be used as preventatives against food poisoning. Sixteen children with Salmonella poisoning and fifteen with Shigella infections were cleared of all symptoms by using acidophilus.[52]

### (8) Inhibit Tumors and Carcinogenesis
Over the last 30 years, several studies have revealed that lactic cultures possess anticarcinogenic properties and are capable of suppressing tumor growth through various mechanisms.[53] The

most effective organism for this purpose is *L. bulgaricus*, but a review of findings from Bulgaria, Denmark, Russia, Japan, and the United States[54] show that antitumor properties have also been credited to special strains of *Bifidobacterium infantis, S. thermophilus, L. acidophilus, L. helveticus, L. casei,* and *L. lactis.*

Hints that lactobacillus can be helpful in treating cancer originated from Bulgaria. In a book published in 1982, Bulgarian physician Ivan Bogdanov discussed his experiences in treating 100 cancer patients with a hydrolyzed extract of *Lactobacillus bulgaricus.* Bogdanov administered the extract orally or intravenously to his patients, who suffered from dozens of types of cancer. In some cases, the extract was given to counter the effects of radiation and chemotherapy; where other therapies had failed, the extract was given alone. Bogdanov stated that the results differed among the patients, ranging from partial remissions to total cures.

Another study revealed that extracts prepared from *L. acidophilus, L. bulgaricus, L. bulgaricus* var. *tumoronecroticans,* and *L. casei* effectively inhibited the growth of sarcoma 180 and Ehrlich carcinoma.[55] In preliminary studies, Reddy et al.[56] observed that mice fed yogurt for 7 days displayed from 28–35 percent inhibition of Ehrlich ascites tumor, a type of cancer.

In another study we examined the effects of feeding and intraperitoneal implantation (planted directly in the stomach) of yogurt culture cells and cell fractions on Ehrlich ascites tumor proliferation. When extracts of probiotic organisms were taken from their cell walls and infused into rats having a variety of tumors, there was a marked (20% or more) reduction in tumor size and growth, and life expectancy of the test animals was twice that of the affected control group.

By inhibiting the growth of putrefactive bacteria, production of N-nitroso compounds, phenolic products of tyrosine and tryptophan, metabolites of biliary steroids, and other potential carcinogens in the colon were reduced.[57]

Further studies have demonstrated that lactobacilli may be involved in repair of the DNA damage caused by nitrosamines in guinea pigs.[58]

## TABLE 1

Effect of feeding lactic acid, fresh milk, fermented milks, fresh colostrum, and fermented colostrum on proliferation of Ehrlich ascites tumor cells

| Material fed | Tumor cells | | Inhibition (%) |
|---|---|---|---|
| | Control | Test | |
| Lactic acid | 28.9 | 32.3 | 0 |
| Fresh milk | 28.9 | 32.3 | 0 |
| Yogurt from milk | 29.5 | 21.4 | 27.4 |
| L. acidophilus milk | 29.2 | 19.8 | 32.1 |
| L. bulgaricus milk | 26.4 | 18.3 | 30.7 |
| Fresh colostrum | 27.2 | 27.4 | 0 |
| Yogurt from colostrum | 32.4 | 23.6 | 27.2 |
| L. acidophilus colostrum | 25.2 | 18.8 | 25.3 |
| L. bulgaricus colostrum | 26.4 | 17.3 | 34.5 |

SOURCE: K. M. Shahani and P. J. Bailey. 1983. "Antitumor activity of fermented colostrum and milk," *J. Food Protect.* 46: 385–386.

The antitumor activity of bifidobacteria is thought to be associated with components of the cell wall.[59]

The author did some collaborative research work with Sloan-Kettering Institute (Rye, New York) and found that the *Lactobacillus acidophilus* DDS-1 strain did tend to retard the growth of certain cancers. There appeared to be a direct relationship between the amount of yogurt consumed and tumor inhibition, and feeding concentrated yogurt also increased inhibition.

In our study performed via the National Dairy Research Institute in India, two groups of six subjects each were used in a switchover experimental design with two treatments (milk and unfermented acidophilus milk).[60] The ingestion of either milk or unfermented acidophilus milk did not have any significant effect on the total aerobic counts in stools. The consumption of acidophilus milk, however, did result in a decrease of the coliform counts. Also significant increases in lactobacillus counts were observed when the diet of the subjects was supplemented with acidophilus milk. The high lactobacillus count was maintained even when acidophilus milk supplementation was discontinued. The ingestion of acidophilus milk instead of milk resulted in a reduced activity of fecal $\beta$-glucosidase and $\beta$-glucuronidase, enzymes which reportedly catalyze the conversion of procarcinogens into carcinogens.[60]

As we know, consumption of lactobacillus products and supplements containing viable lactic acid bacteria results in their establishment in the gastrointestinal tract. Their presence in the intestinal tract has been suggested to be prophylactic. They may reduce risk associated with dietary onset of carcinogenesis directly due to the reduction of procarcinogenic substances or indirectly due to the reduction in the level of enzymes that convert procarcinogens to carcinogens.

The anticarcinogenic property of yogurt microbes and other lactic flora can be classified into three broad categories: elimination of procarcinogens, modulation of procarcinogenic enzymes, and tumor suppression.

*Elimination of procarcinogens*
Nitrites used in food processing are converted to carcinogenic nitrosoamines in the intestinal tract. Cellular uptake of nitrites by lactobacilli results in their chemical and enzymatic depletion. *L. acidophilus* strains can deplete nitrite *in vitro*,[61] but there are differences among strains. However, no information is available on the nitrite depletion mechanism by *L. acidophilus*. Recently, Dodds and Collins-Thompson[62] partially characterized the nitrite reductase activity in *Lactobacillus lactis*. The cellular utilization of nitrites reduces the potential of their conversion to nitrosoamines, eventually reducing the incidence of colon cancer.

*Modulation of procarcinogenic fecal enzymes*
Fecal enzymes (azoreductase, $\beta$-glucuronidase, and nitroreductase) have been used to monitor mucosal carcinogenesis as they convert the procarcinogens to carcinogens.[63, 64] In general, the higher the enzyme level the higher the potential for carcinogenesis. Sinha[65] also observed a decrease in fecal $\beta$-glucuronidase following ingestion of *L. acidophilus*.

Williams et al.[66] as well as Roed and Medtvedt[67] showed that β-glucuronidase activity was primarily of bacterial origin. Kent et al.[68] detected this enzyme in the strictly anaerobic strains belonging to the genera Peptostreptococcus, Corynebacterium, Propionibacterium, Bacteroides, Clostridium, and Cantenabacterium. In contrast, Hawksworth et al.[69] observed a β-glucuronidase activity in both facultative and strictly anaerobic strains belonging to the family *Enterobacteriaceae* and the genera Streptococcus, Lactobacillus, Bifidobacterium, Clostridium, and Bacteroides. Gadeile et al.[70] observed that the β-glucuronidase belonged to three genera Clostridium, Peptostreptococcus, and Staphylococcus. If feeding of *L. acidophilus* cells alters the gastrointestinal microecology favorably and results in a decrease in procarcinogenic enzymes, then the level of these enzymes must be high in undesired fecal flora and low or absent in *L. acidophilus* cells. However, more research needs to be done to examine the presence of β-glucuronidase, azoreductase, and nitroreductase activities among intestinal bacteria.

*Tumor suppression and immune response*
The tumor-suppression property is associated with intact, viable, whole cells[71]; intact dead cells[72]; and cell wall fragments of lactobacilli.[73] Friend et al.[74] observed that the tumor-suppressing agent of *Lactobacillus bulgaricus* was present in the insoluble fraction of sonicated cells (cells broken up by sound waves), but the soluble fraction did not suppress tumor cell proliferation. The antitumor constituent was also associated with the cell wall and the whole cells of *Bifidobacterium infantis*[75, 76] and the insoluble fraction of *Streptococcus thermophilus*. Kohwi et al.[77, 78] found that the cell wall obtained by sonication of killed *B. infantis* suppressed tumors in mice. In contrast, the water-soluble supernatant fraction of these sonicated cells did not suppress tumors. This corroborates the fact that the tumor-suppressing trait was mediated through the bacterial cell wall fraction. Of late there has been considerable interest in the tumor-suppression mechanism by lactobacilli. Antimutagenic tests are also used to study the antitumor properties of substances present in cultured dairy products. Hosono

and Kashina[79] have demonstrated the antimutagenic property of yogurt *in vitro* in Salmonella and *E. coli.*

### (9) Fight Fungal/Yeast/Candida Infections

Studying the antiviral/antifungal properties of various lactic-acid-producing bacteria, Mayer determined that *B. bifidum* was also effective against some viral infections, particularly herpes.[80] *B. bifidum* prevented the overgrowth following penicillin therapy of *Candida albicans*, the most common organism involved in troublesome yeast infections among adults and children. This antifungal activity encouraged Dr. Shahani to study other related organisms. A healthy intestinal population of lactic acid formers, particularly *L. acidophilus*, *B. bifidum*, and *E. faecium*, he found, was effective not only against fungal infections but also against viruses and bacteria. A possible explanation was given by Tihole,[81] who found that lactobacilli are absorbed into the lymphatics where they circulate and cause bacterial and viral-fighting blood cells to be stimulated. For this and other reasons, the authors recommend that the ideal regimen for treating yeast infections includes a supplement containing each of these three organisms.

### (10) Promote or Aid Liver Function and Detoxification

Pollution, toxins in the environment, and ingestion of drugs, alcohol, and food additives place a great strain on the liver and can overload its function of detoxifying the bloodstream.

The bifidobacteria help liver function. For one thing, they detoxify bile, from which they recycle estrogen (a female hormone) in women.[82] This reduces the likelihood of menopausal symptoms and osteoporosis.

### (11) Prevent Osteoporosis

Lack of intake and absorption of dietary calcium is often an important component of osteoporosis. Milk products are a high source of calcium, yet are not easily digested by many people who cannot easily digest lactose. By adding lactic bacteria that produce lactase to the diet, more people are able to tolerate and benefit from the calcium in dairy products. The bacteria also promote the absorption of calcium.

Vitamin K is synthesized by intestinal bacteria, as are the B vitamins, which prevent vitamin K deficiency and aid not only in blood clotting but also in the synthesis of osteocalcin, the protein matrix upon which calcium is crystallized and stored in bone tissue.[83] For this reason, and because lactobacilli enhance calcium assimilation,[84] long-term antibiotic therapy, which kills intestinal bacteria, given without replacement of these bacteria, may contribute to osteoporosis; these bacteria should therefore be included in any program designed to prevent osteoporosis.

### (12) Augment the Immune System

Most of all, the probiotics tend to improve and/or augment the immune responses.[85] It has been documented that lactobacilli may enhance macrophage and lymphocytic activity. This means that the cellular-mediated immune system becomes more powerful and more effective.[86]

Pasteurized yogurt has much less lymphocytic interferon activity than live yogurt. Pasteurized yogurt is yogurt that has been heated; therefore, all the microorganisms in it are dead, and they are not able to exert any effect as do the live organisms in unpasteurized yogurt.[87]

*Streptococcus thermophilus* has been shown to significantly enhance the enzymatic and phagocytic activity of peritoneal macrophages when compared to the control; it also accelerated the function of the reticuloendothelial system as shown by the carbon clearance test.[88]

### (13) Enhance Calcium Assimilation/Metabolism

Bifidobacteria tend to enhance the retention and metabolism of certain minerals, particularly iron and calcium.

Acidophilus or lactic cultures, by virtue of the fact that they produce lactic acid, reduce the pH and thereby increase and enhance the metabolism of calcium and improve absorption.

It has been found that this may reduce the incidence of osteoporosis, hypertension, and cancer.[89]

## (14) Prevent Bad Breath and Flatulence Caused by Intestinal Conditions

Putrefying bacteria that colonize in the gastrointestinal tract, throat, tongue, and mouth cause halitosis.[90] Because they produce natural antibioticlike agents, the probiotics help suppress the proliferation or growth of the bad bacteria, thereby preventing or reducing gas (flatulence), bloating, cramps, and bad breath.[91]

## (15) Promote Human Longevity

In his book *Stay Young*, Ivan Popov, M.D., writes: "Metchnikoff was also one of the first gerontologists (a specialist studying and treating the aging and aged). He maintained that death was not a normal physiologic phenomenon, but a chronic disease against which a remedy could theoretically be found. Gerontology would have progressed more rapidly if Metchnikoff's contributions hadn't been forgotten for a time and, later, rediscovered. . . ."

Metchnikoff was enchanted by the fact that so many people in Bulgarian villages lived beyond 100 years, and he wanted to know why. He found that yogurt was certainly one important reason.

Popov further states that yogurt is effective in curing digestive diseases brought on by too-frequent use of antibiotics, which often destroy intestinal flora. He also mentions that, some years ago, Professor Rene Dubos of Rockefeller University discovered that yogurt not only increases resistance to infection but also prolongs the life span of animals.

## (16) Produce B Vitamins

While many of the lactobacilli require B vitamins for growth, several cultures are capable of synthesizing vitamins. The extent of biosynthesis depends on the temperature, length of incubation, and other processing parameters. Much data is available concerning B-vitamin synthesis by lactobacilli, but very few reports exist on synthesis of vitamins by *L. acidophilus*.

Moreover, there are differences in the methodology of estimating the vitamin levels and enumerating the acidophilus counts, so due consideration must be given when comparing data from various laboratories. Only certain strains from the author's laboratory are known to synthesize B vitamins in special growth media.[92]

*Vitamin Deficiency and Impaired Digestion*
Rao and Shahani determined that cultured dairy products contain a higher concentration of B vitamins than whole cow's milk or mother's milk. The difference is attributed to *L. acidophilus* and other lactobacilli, which steadily synthesize B vitamins, especially folic acid and biotin. This constant provision of B vitamins through lactobacilli helps prevent a vitamin B deficiency and facilitates food digestion, partly because B vitamins are biocatalysts and thereby increase digestive enzyme activity.[93]

Niacin, pantothenic acid, pyridoxine, $B_6$, and $B_{12}$ are also manufactured by probiotics.

## (17) Synthesize Vitamin K
One of the key vitamins synthesized by acidophilus in the intestines is vitamin K, which helps blood to clot. When a person fails to have sufficient bacteria in the colon—or fails to derive it from food or to take a vitamin K supplement—osteocalcin cannot be properly formed.[94]

So what is osteocalcin and why is it so important? Osteocalcin enables calcium to be crystallized and transported into the bones. Without sufficient osteocalcin, one is an excellent candidate for developing osteoporosis.

## (18) Reduce pH
Lactic cultures of the probiotics reduce pH by virtue of the fact that they produce lactic and other acids.

## (19) Protect Against Numerous Disease Conditions
Probiotics play a fundamental role (in conjunction with other lifestyle considerations) in protecting patients from a multitude of disease conditions; bacterial, viral, and fungal infections; heart disease, osteoporosis, allergy, dermatitis, anxiety, and various cancers, particularly colon cancer.

A deficiency (imbalance) sets the stage for a cascade of events that may lead to the onset and progression of these and many other disease conditions.

Although these microorganisms are not by themselves a cure-all, doctors of every specialty will clearly benefit from a better understanding of their functions, knowing the food sources in which they are found, discerning the need to choose supplements carefully, and discovering how the use of these organisms might enhance a patient's treatment outcome—no matter what the problem is.[95]

### (20) Improve General Gastrointestinal Health and Prevent Disorders

The probiotics play an important part of the development of a baby's digestive function and immune system. When the *Bifidobacterium infantis*, which should be acquired from breast milk is lacking or in poor supply, allergies and malabsorption problems are common.[96]

German research shows that the intestinal flora in most breast-fed babies today is similar to that of formula-fed babies 40 years ago. The result is malabsorption and food sensitivity problems, as well as allergies and susceptibility to infection. This suggests that supplementation of all babies with bifidobacterium may be a helpful strategy.

In addition, balanced flora play a critical role in the prevention of bowel irregularity.

The number of beneficial intestinal and vaginal microorganisms decreases with the increasing uses of antibiotics and other drugs, resulting in constipation, diarrhea, vaginitis, and other health problems that generally do not develop when *L. acidophilus* and other helpful bacteria are in strong supply.[97]

Marvin Speck, Ph.D., from North Carolina State University stated that the antibiotic therapy that causes intestinal distress often coincides with the reduction or elimination of lactobacilli in the feces. The coliform or other pathogens are then able to proliferate and produce acids and gas that result in diarrhea and flatulence. Ingesting lactobacilli reestablishes the normal balance of the intestinal microflora and brings relief from the intestinal distress.[98]

Many of the strains of good bacteria available in supplement form work to support healthy bowel ecology. One strain in particular that has been receiving quite a bit of attention lately is *Lactobacillus salivarius*. A friendly bacteria that scientists have known about for almost 100 years, *L. salivarius* has only recently been stabilized for use as a supplement. The bacteria is said to perform a very important and useful role in the body.

It is very active on proteins as well as by-products of protein putrefaction. This allows the bacteria to accomplish the breakdown of undigested proteins, making nutrition readily available to the body while rendering pathogenic toxins inert.

This friendly bacteria combined with other bacteria, like acidophilus and bifidus mentioned earlier, offer tremendous support for good colon health.[99]

Several studies have shown the following:

- Milk soured when *L. bulgaricus* was fed to subjects with intestinal putrefaction; putrefaction decreased and stools became normal, predominately with Gram-positive flora.[100]

- Yogurt helped restore the normal intestinal flora previously disturbed by antibiotic therapy.[101]

- Children suffering from infantile diarrhea recovered more rapidly when fed yogurt than did those given neomycin—Kaopectate.[102]

- *L. acidophilus* could be used to maintain a stable, protective intestinal flora while pathogenic organisms were being eliminated.[103]

- The administration of acidophilus reduced the number of intestinal *E. coli* substantially, and the flora in stools consisted almost entirely of *L. acidophilus*.[104]

- The administration of yogurt or modified yogurt alleviated significantly the chronic constipation of geriatrics, as well as improved the general health, skin tone, and chronic intestinal disturbance.[105, 106]

Dr. Walter Schmidt has found clinically that burning symptoms anywhere in the body are often an indication of colon floral imbalance.[107] This is especially true of burning feet, which may also be related to Thiamine (vitamin $B_1$) deficiency, or the more severe problem of diabetic neuropathy, and therefore this symptom deserves careful differential diagnosis whenever it is encountered.[108]

### (21) Contribute to Radiation Protection

The bifidobacteria prevent potential toxicity from nitrates in food.[109] In a study with guinea pigs, it was noted that irradiation of the experimental group of animals receiving acidophilus milk did not cause abnormalities in their offspring. Also, offspring developed better and gained more weight than those from an untreated control group of guinea pigs that had not received acidophilus milk.[110]

### (22) Retard or Prevent Dermatological (Skin) Problems

Therapeutically, probiotics have been shown to be useful in treatment of acne, psoriasis, eczema, and other skin conditions.

*L. acidophilus* helps alleviate dermatitis and other skin disorders by modifying and improving gastrointestinal microbial balance.

In some patients with atopic eczema, severely disturbed balances of intestinal microflora can cause itching and depressed immune function. But researchers in the Spezial Klinik Neukirchen in Germany, led by Dr. Gruia Ionescu, found that the most consistent finding among eczema patients was absence of (or dramatically reduced) lactobacilli, and that these symptoms are greatly alleviated after a 10-week course of *L. acidophilus* supplements.[111]

Recurrent problems with skin fungus such as athletes foot (especially in children) are frequently accompanied by large intestine floral imbalance. The quality of the perspiration of the feet (and other skin areas as well) is affected by the imbalance of intestinal flora. The bowel and the skin are both organs of elimination and thereby affect each other.[112]

## (23) Therapeutically Benefit Arthritic Conditions

Rheumatoid arthritis and ankylosing spondylitis have been found to be associated with overgrowth in the intestines of particular harmful bacteria, Proteus and Klebsiella, respectively.[113] Both of these can be controlled by healthy bowel flora. The natural antibioticlike substances manufactured by *Lactobacillus bulgaricus*, *Lactobacillus acidophilus*, and the bifidobacteria kill both of these bacteria.[114]

British research shows that people with ankylosing spondylitis benefit if they go on a diet low in fat and sugar and high in complex carbohydrates, the very diet that enables friendly bacteria to perform efficiently.

In recent Norwegian trials, rheumatoid arthritis patients have been shown to benefit from a vegetarian diet, which also dramatically improves the health and function of the friendly bacteria.[115]

## (24) Prevent and Control Diarrhea

An alternative to antibiotics has been examined in order to provide a useful first-choice treatment of enteritis, and antibiotics are being reserved for only those clinical conditions where the etiological bacterial agent is known.

*Enterococcus faecium* has been used by Underdahl[116] and Lewenstein et al.[117] in the treatment of diarrheal diseases in animals and humans, respectively. In gnotobiotic pigs (pigs with a sterile gut), challenged with *E. coli* alone and in combination with *E. faecium*, Underdahl observed that the diarrheal state was reversed in two days, and the pigs fed *Enterococcus faecium* gained more weight than the control group that was challenged with only *E. coli*.

Lewenstein et al.[117] carried out a preliminary clinical observation on 14 in-patients (11 men and 3 women, aged 22 to 82 years) who were suffering from different diarrheal disorders. Patients were given 3 or 4 capsules a day during a 6- to 10-day period without any other therapy except dietary prescriptions or rehydration and occasional antispasmodic drugs, if necessary.

# Probiotics and Stress

Ongoing research is revealing the intimate connection between our body's response to stress and the healthy balance of our gut bacteria. Evidence from this research mounts that prolonged stress responses can shift the balance of friendly bacteria toward more pathogenic species. Other research indicates that a healthy balance of friendly bacteria can shield us from otherwise powerful stressors in our environment. Both point generally toward prophylactic probiotic ingestion as a stress buffer in our complex and often toxic world.

## Psychological Stress

In a study by Baily and Coe of the University of Wisconsin Department of Psychology abstracted in the *Journal of Neuroimmunomodulation* (Vol. 6, 1999), infant rhesus monkeys separated from their mothers were shown to have increased pathogenic bacteria and infections, presumably due to the psychological stress of this separation. The authors of the study conclude: "These results demonstrate that strong emotional reactions to disruption of the mother-infant bond can disrupt the integrity of the indigenous microflora, resulting in an intestinal environment conducive to pathogen colonization and proliferation."

## Radiation Stress

Edward Block, Ph.D., in his book, *For the Life in Your Food!* (1999) sites clinical research performed upon Japanese survivors of the atomic blasts in Hiroshima and Nagasaki as a prime example of the ability of friendly microflora to buffer the harmful effects of stressful radiation exposure. Based on interviews by U.S. medical personnel, most of the long-term survivors acknowledged eating a traditional Japanese diet while most of the short-term survivors preferred consuming a preponderance of Western foods. The Japanese diet emphasized naturally fermented and pickled foods containing an abundance of friendly microorganisms: *Lactobacillus acidophilus, Propionbacter sp., Pseudomonas sp., Acetobacter sp., Pediococcus pentosaceus* and *halophilus, Aspergillus orzae* and *soyae, Saccharomyces sp.,* and *Candida versatilis.* Dr. Blocks concludes that the basis for this radiation hardiness was that

"These microorganisms conferred survivability due to the fact that they kept harmful bacteria from growing in the damaged alimentary tract."

### Athletic Stress

According to researchers Chen, Zhao and Qioa, in a study reported in the *Hong Kong Journal of Sports Medicine and Sports* (Volume XV, November 2002), gastrointestinal (GI) problems are extremely common among athletes. Symptoms include nausea, bloating, heartburn, acid reflux, diarrhea, the urge to defecate, and rectal bleeding. The dynamics of intestinal microflora are regarded as an "important factor" in causing these GI problems by these researchers. Further sports research in two studies now being conducted in Germany shows likely immunostimulatory effects of probiotic supplementation on athletes given a probiotic blend during post-exercise periods of immunosuppression. In the growing field of Sports Medicine and Nutrition, this recent research confirms the promising role of probiotics in the health and performance of athletes.

### Toxic Metal Stress

In an article published in the *Indian Journal of Medical Research* (Vol. 119, Feb. 2004, pp. 49–59, authored by Upreti, Shrivastava, and Chaturvedi), the role of gut microflora in relationship to heavy metal detoxification was examined using chromium as a model. Although the precise mechanism remains unclear, the article states that a population of healthy bacteria in the gut serves to sequester and reduce the levels of toxic chromium in the system (and other toxic metals as well). The researchers conclude that "resident gut microflora plays a very important role in protection against metal toxicity."

### Emotional Stress

In an article published in the *Journal of Clinical Nutrition* (1978; 31: S33–S42), the role of emotional stress upon the intestinal microflora was examined. Moore et al reported "the composition of the flora was not significantly affected by drastic changes in diet, but statistically significant shifts in the proportion of some species [beneficial to harmful] were noted in individuals under conditions of anger or fear stress."

They observed that the diarrhea and abdominal pain, which were very strong during the start of the treatment, disappeared in all cases after one to three days. The starting pH values of the feces ranged from 7.5 to 8.5 and fell to 7.0 in 2 to 3 days. The ratio of Gram-negative to Gram-positive flora reached normalcy in 2 to 4 days. The enteropathogenic *E. coli* was never detected in the cultures of the feces after only 2 days of treatment. No abnormality was detected in blood chemistry examination.

Lewenstein et al.[117] found that the biological and microbiological properties of the *Enterococcus faecium* makes it suitable for use in diarrhea disturbances. Particularly in cases where pathogenic microbes invade the bowel, resulting in a disturbed biological balance of the intestinal flora, *Enterococcus faecium* is an excellent candidate because of its special properties: intestinal commensal (naturally found in the intestines), a brief period between introduction and fast growth, short generation time, strong inhibitory effect on growth of *E. coli* and Salmonella *in vitro*, production of lactic acid, resistance to many chemotherapeutic drugs, lack of pathogenicity, and high tolerability without side effects.

*Enterococcus faecium* is a normal inhabitant of the gastrointestinal tract of man and animals. This organism is a lactic acid producer and has shown some promising biological properties for clinical therapeutic use in veterinary medicine. *Enterococcus faecium* was first classified as *Streptoccus faecium*, but it was reclassified because of special biochemical reactions. Now it has been renamed officially *Enterococcus faecium*.

During diarrhea symptoms, the intestinal microecology gets out of balance. In such a diseased state, antibiotics are administered. Antibiotics themselves cause diarrhea and consequently alter the gut microbiota, resulting in proliferation and inhabitation of drug-resistant microbes. Thus it is essential to treat these symptoms with care without changing the microbial environment of the gastrointestinal tract.

Following the consumption of cultured dairy products, lactobacillus, or other lactic-acid-producing bacteria, an alteration in the intestinal microflora occurs, particularly an increase in the lactobacillus population, as observed in the feces.[118] This alteration is probably due to the antimicrobial substances produced by lactic-acid-producing bacteria, or due to the overpowering effect of these organisms. Lactic-acid-producing bacteria would be most effective when the number of invading pathogenic bacteria is relatively small. Also, these bacteria would most likely be effective when they are present in the gastrointestinal tract prior to infection, and therefore may prevent the invading pathogenic bacteria from colonizing. The evidence reviewed here indicates to us that lactic-acid-producing bacteria have potential not only in the prevention of diarrhea, but also for its therapy.

The control of infant and adult diarrhea by lactobacilli has been attempted in recent years with much success. *B. bifidum*, *Enterococcus faecium*, and *L. acidophilus* are most effective in correcting infant diarrhea; *L. acidophilus* and *E. faecium* are effective in correcting adult diarrhea. Even nonfermented acidophilus milk appears to have a positive effect on infant diarrhea, prompting researchers to conclude that even simple dietary improvements involving probiotic supplementation, without antibiotic therapy, can be effective.[119]

For infant diarrhea, the standard remedy includes oral administration of *B. bifidum* in human milk, cream of rice cereal, some electrolytes, and a high-fluid diet. For adult diarrhea, the recommendation is for 3–4 capsules daily of a supplement containing *B. bifidum* taken for 6–10 days, and sufficient liquids to rehydrate.[120]

In the early or middle 1980s, it was observed in Bangladesh that diarrhea was so rampant that "a child died every 6 seconds, 10 every minute, 600 every hour." Research work for the World Health Organization (WHO) of the United Nations and the International Center for Diarrheal Disease Research, Bangladesh (ICDDRB) showed that diarrhea could be effectively controlled by administering *E. faecium* coupled with a rice oral rehydration solution containing electrolytes.[121]

In summary, the ability of intestinal flora to metabolize nutrients, hormones, bile acids, cholesterol, and carcinogens is well established. We are just beginning to learn about how the bacteria that reside in our gut impact human metabolism and health, as well as what potential impact a deficiency has on these organisms.

## *Summary of Probiotic Health Benefits*

- Promoting a well-functioning gastrointestinal system

- Replacing friendly flora destroyed by antibiotics

- Maintaining the natural balance of internal physiological functions in our body

- Supporting the beneficial microorganisms in the gut that prevent or reduce the effects of infectons caused by pathogens

- Metabolizing the food we eat and living symbiotically with our bodies, performing many life-supporting functions

"When I was growing up my Dad, a dentist, used to take jars of my mother's homemade yogurt to his patients who were on antibiotics. This simple introduction of helpful bacteria prevented all manner of side effects.

I have carried on my father's wise practice for 25 years in my work in women's health. I consider probiotics one of the most useful—and underutilized—modalities available for preserving health."

Christiane Northrup
Author, *Women's Bodies, Women's Wisdom* (Bantam 1998)
and *The Wisdom of Menopause* (Bantam 2001)

# The Candida Epidemic

## *Fighting Yeast Infections*

Yeasts are all around us—in the soil, on our food, in the water, and, yes, in our bodies. The truth is, yeast is essential to life and good health![1]

*Candida albicans* and *Candida parapsilosis* are two of several yeast (fungal) organisms normally present in the human body. These organisms have been around for thousands of years, living symbiotically within man, and, yes, they are good guys to have around—in appropriate quantities and in balance with the natural ecosystem of the human body.

Candidiasis refers to a parasitic infection (usually with *Candida albicans* and/or *parapsilosis*) whereby levels of these yeasts increase dramatically, well beyond acceptable, ecologically balanced levels.[2]

Candida has a visible life cycle: It advances from a normal nonpathogenic form and literally evolves into an abnormal pathogenic form.[3] Normally, these candida fungi reside naturally as part of normal body flora in the mouth, gastrointestinal tracts, skin, and vaginal cavities, where other friendly bacteria help the immune system keep the proper balance of organisms, including candida, under control.

In these modern times, this proper balance has not always been kept in check. Candida has, in fact, overtaken the health of many whose immunity has been compromised.

Diets rich in sugar, cortisone and cortisonelike drugs, birth control pills, immuno-suppressive drugs and antibiotics (the "double-edged sword"), have been major culprits in the "candida epidemic" of today.

A number of immunologists suggest that the health of approximately 80 million Americans may be adversely affected by candidiasis.[4]

Vaginal Candidiasis (Monila) usually follows antibiotic therapy or when the immune system is otherwise suppressed.[5]

Oral Candidiasis (Thrush) is found mostly in babies, but sometimes in older children or adults, when the body's resistance is worn down. Bottle-fed infants, those using unsanitary bottle nipples, those on antibiotic and other drug therapy, or those suffering from poor nutrition may, in their weakened condition, develop Thrush.[6]

Candidiasis (excess colonization) in the intestinal tract can occur if the normal bacterial flora is suppressed by antibiotics, chemotherapy, or poor nutrition.

Respiratory candidiasis may develop in people with severe respiratory problems (pneumonia, chronic bronchitis, etc.); they are usually taking strong drugs, especially antibiotics, that interfere with the immune responses.[7]

Candidiasis on the skin occurs if a person is very ill and has suffered injury to the skin. Internal antibiotics promote this condition also.[8]

Systemic candidiasis (i.e., where candida spreads throughout the entire body) may occur in a person who is severely immune compromised, such as a person with AIDS or cancer.[9]

It has been stated, and the author agrees, that fungus (like candidiasis) poses mankind's greatest health challenge today—it is mankind's greatest threat. Time to listen up!

Candida is a single-celled organism. It reproduces asexually and thrives on the body's by-products: dead tissue and sugars from food. Candidiasis develops when there is an unnatural balance in the body. A deficiency of healthy bacteria may lead to yeast overgrowth. Often this deficiency was caused by antibiotics, which rapidly destroy the beneficial bacteria.[10]

Many people are unaware that they consume antibiotics daily, without a doctor's prescription, in the food they eat. Antibiotics are routinely used as supplements in animal feed or in the treatment of sick livestock. As a result, humans who eat these types of animal products that contain antibiotics may be destroying their native bacteria and paving the way for fungal overgrowth.

This fungal overgrowth creates a vicious cycle because yeasts consume valuable nutrients, such as the B vitamins, which are desperately needed by the tissues. This in turn leads to more tissue degradation, which in turn leads to more by-products for the yeasts to feast on. This intestinal imbalance is similar to what we may refer to as interfering with ecological balance in the external world.

If man destroys too many of a certain species of an animal, for instance, then an insect that this animal normally eats can become overpopulated, causing more and more harm. Allowing the animals to again increase to normal numbers eliminates the problem with the insects, and the balance is restored.

So too with candidiasis! The natural restoration of this biological balance to the human body must include several definite factors:

1. Elimination of harmful antibiotics and drugs.
2. Elimination of destructive stressors on the body.
3. Reduction of sugar from refined foods (candida's favorite).
4. Elimination of allergenic foods, as these place stress on the immune system.
5. Restoration and continual replenishment of the body with all its basic nutrient needs in high quality forms: adequate oxygen, water, fiber, vitamins, minerals, enzymes, proteins, fats, and complex carbohydrates.
6. Replenishment of adequate probiotic flora.

In his book entitled *The Yeast Connection*, Dr. William Crook summarizes very succinctly the noted efficacy of acidophilus and supplement preparations against yeast-related disorders.

Further work in our laboratory has shown that by proper growing and incubation techniques, the genetic composition of *L. acidophilus* can be changed, which then augments the immune bodies of the consumers.[11]

Often we are impressed with how fast antibiotics can kill harmful microorganisms. As Dr. Shahani has shown, antibiotic-like substances called bacteriocins, which he has produced in milk by means of fermentation using *L. acidophilus*, can be even more potent. The agent acidophilin packs more killing power than penicillin, streptomycin, or teramycin. The killing power of acidophilus is not limited to its antibiotic effect. It annihilates disease-causing microorganisms with other biochemical weapons: acetic acid, benzoic acid, hydrogen peroxide, and lactic acid.

Acidophilus, on its own or in yogurt, has developed a reputation for defeating long-standing yeast infections. A single cup of yogurt a day reduced vaginitis threefold in women with recurrent candida overgrowth, as discovered by Eileen Hilton, M.D., of Long Island Jewish Medical Center in New York, who studied 16 women over 12 months.[12]

In a study involving 30 women at the University of California at Davis, Edwin B. Collins, Ph.D., and colleagues reported in the *Journal of Dairy Science* that *L. acidophilus* produces metabolites that inhibit *Candida albicans,* which causes painful yeast infections such as monilia vaginitis.

As reported in *Lancet,* 20 women with candida vulvovaginitis were cured with preparations containing *L. acidophilus.*[13]

In studying 12 patients with Gardnerella-associated vaginitis, Fredricsson et al. reported that significantly larger numbers of lactobacilli were present in the vagina when the patients were symptom-free.[14]

"I take acidophilus with meals when I travel in under-developed countries," said Andrew Weil, M.D., in *Natural Health, Natural Medicine.* "I believe it reduced the chance of getting traveler's diarrhea, the result of changes in intestinal flora. I recommend acidophilus to anyone who takes antibiotics, especially the broad-spectrum ones like tetracycline and ampicillin, which wreak havoc on intestinal floras. I recommend it also to women who have frequent vaginal yeast infections. The dose is one tablespoon of the liquid culture or one or two capsules after meals unless the label directs otherwise. To treat yeast infection, you can also place the liquid culture directly in the vagina in addition to taking it by mouth."

In addition to acidophilus, Dr. Weil recommends that women who are prone to vaginal yeast infections should reduce their sugar intake and add raw garlic to their diets.

In addition to antibiotics, oral contraceptives, aspirin, corticosteroids, poor diet, some kinds of yeast, and stress all contribute to candidiasis, according to James F. Balch, M.D., and Phyllis A. Balch, in *Prescription for Nutritional Health.* The beneficial bacteria bind with some of the unwanted substances and are excreted.

For those suffering from allergies, the Balches recommend milk-free acidophilus products, which are especially useful against candida infections. Since some of the products use carrot juice as a base, they are ideal for vegetarians or others who do not use milk products.[15]

The nondairy forms of acidophilus have antifungal properties, reduce blood cholesterol levels, aid digestion, and enhance absorption of nutrients, according to the Balches.[15]

In addition to oral use of probiotics for vaginal yeast infections, it is recommended that 2–3 capsules of a probiotic that includes acidophilus be inserted into the vagina each night. These infections can be very difficult to overcome. Because the body is less stressed during sleep, a woman will receive maximum benefit during this time.

Put simply, the destructive substances and stressors must be eliminated and the body's cells, tissues, and organs must continually get what they need to support their life. Also, there must be continual proper elimination of the waste matter, or fungus can take its opportunity and monopolize entire body cells, organs, and systems.

According to the prominent German physician Dr. Enderlein, it is necessary to address both the causative microorganism and to change the body's internal environment to cure the illness—candidiasis.[16]

To improve their inner ecology and restore a proper pH balance, it is recommended that candida patients make the proper dietary changes and avoid unnecessary burdening of the body with antibiotics and other harmful substances. Incorporating a good exercise program into the lifestyle is also suggested to give the lymphatic system adequate circulation so the body may heal.[17]

## On Probiotics from *What Doctors Don't Tell You* (UK)

**Volume: 12  Issue: 3  Section: Special Report**

### TREATMENT ALTERNATIVES    LYME DISEASE

Alternative medicine has not been proven particularly successful at treating chronic and severe Lyme disease. However, there are several things you can do to support your system as it fights the infection while taking conventional treatment. Watch out for Candida. Patients being treated with antibiotics can develop a yeast overgrowth. To combat this, take two high-quality probiotics after each meal and follow a strict anti-Candida diet, which contains no sugars. If you can tolerate dairy, you may include live yoghurt daily in your diet.

**Volume: 9  Issue: 9  Section: Special Report**

### CANDIDA    NEW THEORIES, NEW CURES (Tony Edwards)

Over the years, conventional antifungals, such as nystatin, have gradually tended to fall out of favor. An increasing number of practitioners are now turning towards natural therapies. First and foremost are the "probiotics." These are specially cultured bacteria, identical to the ones in the gut that normally keep the *C albicans* yeast under control. Once the candida has been cleared by diet or drugs, probiotics are prescribed to repopulate the gut.

Chief among these are species of Lactobacillus and Bifidobacteria (see box, p 2). Apart from competing with *C albicans* for space, they have also been shown to increase intestinal acidity, creating a less favorable environment for candida. Probiotics can be taken either as dry capsules or liquid yoghurts. Although the anecdotal evidence for their effectiveness is overwhelming, there have been few clinical trials for their use in candidiasis.

A recent year-long, crossover trial on *candida vaginitis*, however, showed a threefold decrease in symptoms in patients who ate yoghurt containing *Lactobacillus acidophilus* (*Annals of Internal Medicine*, 1992; 116: 353–7).

**Volume: 8  Issue: 5  Section: Special Report**

### LEAKY GUT    REPAIRING OUR PROTECTIVE FENCE (Leo Galland)

One of the most overlooked causes of disease is not just what we eat but how well we digest it, particularly in our small intestine.

Think of your gut as a one-way fence. The lining of the gut is permeable, that is, small particles of food are able to pass through it into the other cells of our body, but in a healthy body these "holes" are small enough to keep contained molecules which might otherwise cause harm. . . .

Changing the flora of the gut through the use of antibiotics, synthetic and natural, probiotics such as acidophilus (the "friendly bacteria"), and diet is one strategy for breaking the vicious cycle in leaky gut syndromes. Usually, patients whose arthritis is alleviated by a vegetarian diet are those where the diet alters gut ecology; if the diet doesn't do this in a particular case, the arthritis usually isn't improved (*Br J Rheumatol*, 1994; 33: 638–43).

This article was adapted and excerpted from a paper which first appeared in *Townsend Letter for Doctors and Patients* (911 Tyler Street, Port Townsend, WA 98368-6541; Tel: 360-385-6021).

**Source: www.wddty.com**

## Excerpted from Proof! *What Works in Alternative Medicine* (UK)

**Volume: 7  Issue: 12  Section: Newsbits**

*Beneficial bacteria  Adults with ulcerative colitis (UC) may have up to 63 percent fewer flare-ups by taking a fermented-milk supplement (containing at least 10 billion organisms per bottle of *Bifido-bacterium breve*, *B. bifidum*, and *Lactobacillus acidophilus*) (*J Am Coll Nutr*, 2003; 22: 56–63).

*Diet may protect women against urinary tract infections  Women who frequently consume berry juices or fermented-milk products containing probiotics may reduce their risk of recurrent urinary tract infections (UTIs) (*Am J Clin Nutr*, 2003; 77: 600–4).

**Volume: 4  Issue: 1  Section: Cover story**

**Alternative Antibiotics**    Fighting infections naturally (Pat Thomas)

Prevention is better than cure. The stronger your immune system is, the less likely it is that you will succumb to any kind of bug. To prevent bacteria from taking hold or to limit the damage it can cause if it does take hold, consider the following:

. . . If you do take antibiotics:

*Take plenty of probiotics. While you are taking antibiotics and for a time afterwards, make sure you take high levels of bifidobacteria, lactobacilli, FOS or soil-based microorganisms, which will feed and replace friendly bacteria destroyed by the antibiotics.

**Volume: 3  Issue: 2  Section: Laboratory test**

### Probiotics: Who are the big hitters?

Probiotics consist of specially cultured bacteria that are near-identical to the "friendly" bugs that colonize your gut and are present in live yoghurt. These supplements aim to repopulate a gut depleted of the right bacteria through a *Candida albicans* yeast overgrowth, parasitic infection, or other gut disorders. Healthy intestinal "flora," as these bacteria are also called, aid digestion and absorption of food, increase intestinal acidity, and keep unfriendly guests like Candida yeast and other, anaerobic, "bad" bacteria in check. In a normal gut, "good" bacteria will attach themselves to the gut wall and consume any yeasts passing by.

Chief among the "good" bacteria contained in these supplements are *Lactobacillus acidophilus*, your intestine's chief of police, although many products now come with an exotic range of Lactobacillus and Bifidobacterium species, which are also present, in varying amounts, in the gut. *Lactobacillus acidophilus* and *L. bulgaricus*, for instance, mostly reside in the small intestine, while *Bifidobacterium bifidum* largely resides in the large intestine. Most versions come in either a tablet or capsule, but all contain freeze-dried bacteria, which then must be "reconstituted" before going to work in your intestines. . . .

Dr Nigel Plummer, a UK expert on lactic acid bacteria, recommends that any good probiotic supplement should:
* contain at least 1 billion viable cells per daily dose
* include an expiry date
* contain human *L. acidophilus* and bifidobacteria
* be able to tolerate stomach acid and bile (many can't)
* be capable of colonizing the human intestine.

Source: www.wddty.com

# Lactose Intolerance

## *A Global Phenomenon*

The terms *lactase deficiency, lactose intolerance, lactose malabsorption,* and *milk intolerance* have often been used interchangeably. The usage of these terms to describe the hereditary, age-related decrease in lactose digestion capacity has created much confusion. Low lactase activity can be broadly categorized as three main types: congenital lactase deficiency (*Alactasia*), primary adult lactase deficiency (*Hypolactasia*), and secondary lactase deficiency.

Congenital lactase deficiency is an extremely rare occurrence, where lactase is missing throughout life, although the histology of the intestinal mucosa is normal. Primary adult lactase deficiency refers to the normal developmental, age-related decrease in lactose-digesting capacity. In 70 percent of the world's adult population, intestinal lactase activity is low, and this low activity is considered normal. Therefore, it has been recommended that primary adult lactase deficiency be renamed "lactase nonpersistence" and that "lactase persistence" be used to describe individuals who retain abundant intestinal lactase as an autosomal dominant trait. Secondary lactase deficiency is a transient state of low lactase in previously lactase-persistent individuals, following injury to the small intestinal mucosa from diseases such as celiac sprue, infectious gastroenteritis, or protein-energy malnutrition. It is now recommended that secondary lactase deficiency by renamed *lactase deficiency*.

*Lactose malabsorption* implies the incomplete digestion of lactose, resulting in a flat or low rise in blood sugar following a lactose tolerance test. It reflects the outcome but not the cause of the condition. Lactose malabsorption is not a unique reflection of an individual's lactase status, as some gastrointestinal states also can cause lactose malabsorption without decrease in lactose-hydrolyzing capacity.

## TABLE 2

With the exception of the population of Northern and Central Europe and its offspring in America and Austrailia, 70–100% of adults worldwide are lactose malabsorbers.

| Population area | Prevalence of primary lactose maldigestion (%) |
|---|---|
| Africa* | 70–90 |
| Austria | 15–20 |
| Balkans | 55 |
| Central Asia | 80 |
| Eastern Asia | 90–100 |
| Finland | 17 |
| France (northern) | 17 |
| France (southern) | 65 |
| Germany | 15 |
| Great Britain | 5–15 |
| India (northern) | 30 |
| India (southern) | 70 |
| Italy | 20–70 |
| North America (Blacks) | 80 |
| North America (Hispanics) | 53 |
| North America (Caucasians) | 15 |
| Scandinavia | 3–5 |
| South America | 65–75 |

*Exceptions: Tuareg, 13%, Fulani, 22%; Bedouins, 25%*

SOURCE: Statistics from the Institute of Physiology and Biochemistry of Nutrition, Federal Dairy Research Center; Kiel, Germany. Presented at the symposium "Probtiotics and Prebiotics" held in Kiel, Germany, June 11–12, 1998.

*Lactose intolerance* is defined as the occurrence of clinical signs (diarrhea, bloating, flatulence), or subjective symptoms (abdominal pain, gaseousness), following intake of lactose for a standard lactose intolerance test in a person with proven lactose malabsorption.

Bifidobacteria are unique in that all the lactic acid produced is in the L(+) form. L(+) lactic acid is easily metabolized by infants, whereas D(−) lactic acid, produced by *L. acidophilus* and *L. bulgaricus,* can cause metabolic acidosis during the first year of development.

Specifically, lactose maldigestion is the result of insufficient amounts of $\beta$-galactosidase in the human small intestine to digest the milk sugar, lactose. Although normal yogurt cultures *L. bulgaricus* and *S. thermophilus* contain substantial amounts of $\beta$-galactosidase, the enzyme is affected by bile.

Because bifidobacteria are resistant to bile, they may have a better chance of colonizing the gut and delivering their lactose-metabolizing enzymes to the site of action over an extended period of time.[1]

## *Probiotics for the Lactose Intolerant*

Lactose intolerance applies to individuals who have an absent or diminished capacity to produce lactase, the enzyme that hydrolyzes lactose, the milk sugar, into glucose and galactose.

In 1983–84, Nebraska Cultures, formerly known as American Cultures and Enzyme Systems Incorporated, was perhaps the first organization to develop true nondairy and hypoallergenic probiotic cultures. This amazing breakthrough culture contained *Lactobacillus acidophilus* DDS-1 without the use of any dairy-related ingredients.

Today, on the market, probiotics come in powder, tablet, and capsule forms, and in dairy-derived and dairy-free versions. One may encounter various brands of dairy-free probiotics, but the DDS-1 strain is still the most substantially peer-reviewed in the research on this subject.

For true nondairy probiotics suitable for lactose-intolerant/milk-protein-intolerant individuals, look for a scientifically proven dairy-free or nondairy strain.

# Are All Probiotics Alike?

## *Research on* L. acidophilus *and Other Probiotics*

The literature is filled with studies concerning the beneficial role of lactobacilli in general and *L. acidophilus* in particular. Nevertheless, there exist numerous reports indicating divergent and sometimes conflicting observations. It has been established that such conflicting results may very well be due to the different strains used, different manufacturing or propagation methods employed, and, of course, the different techniques used by scientists.

At the University of Nebraska, research on *Lactobacillus acidophilus* was started as early as 1925. The author, Dr. Khem Shahani, initiated his own research around 1958 when he saw that getting the benefits of these flora from both foods and supplements was difficult at best. He felt compelled to find the very best strains, as well as new and superior growth and preservation techniques to ensure successful colonization of beneficial flora in the body. In the development process, he addressed the most critical issues: stability, bioactivity of the flora cells, viability, resistance to digestive activity and antibiotic agents, and, above all, successful implantation in the system.

Since 1958, scientists headed by the author have worked on *L. acidophilus*, *L. bifidus* (renamed *Bifidobacterium bifidum*), and other lactic cultures and have published more than 200 scientific papers on these cultures. They have demonstrated conclusively that considerable differences exist among different strains of *L. acidophilus*. In fact, the same strain grown under different conditions would show different properties.

DDS-1—THE FRIENDLIEST FLORA

Through his research work, the author has optimized exceptional strains of microorganisms, the most noted of which is the extraordinary DDS-1 Acidophilus. This strain of *L. acidophilus* has been extensively researched at the University of Nebraska.

A specially isolated and cultured strain of *L. acidophilus* DDS-1, grown and produced under specific conditions, has properties of great significance for digestion and nutrition and for physiological health and disease.

Dr. Shahani's special methods are exclusive to only a few flora products that are among only a select number of products manufactured at a facility associated with a university research program. This makes DDS-1 *L. acidophilus* unquestionably the finest flora ever produced.

The question often raised in the scientific circles is whether the consumer actually gets the same nutritional and therapeutic benefits from different products that are being marketed.

Each microbe is like an individual and has its own distinct personality. Affection and warmth are given to these microbes through nourishment and temperature. These personality traits can be severely affected if the environment in which they are produced is not conducive to growth. For instance, considerable variations are encountered when cultures are grown at higher than their optimal temperature. Drug resistance is mediated through plasmids, and when bacterial cultures are grown at 46–49°C, some of the drug-resistant plasmids are lost, rendering the strain susceptible to drugs.[1]

All acidophilus products available commercially are not pre-pared alike. The name on the bottle is meaningless if the bottle does not contain the right acidophilus strain. Many cannot even survive stomach fluids. Many products contain extremely low levels of living *L. acidophilus* cells and unstable cells as well. Some manufacturers give numbers of live cells at the time of formula-tion, packaging, or bottling, but after manufacturing and storage, the number of live cells can drop to almost zero.

During the past 20 years or so, as a part of an ongoing research program on probiotics at the University of Nebraska, more than 200 acidophilus products collected from the United States and abroad were examined. Almost 70 to 80 percent of the samples did not measure up to numerical claims and, in fact, nearly 50 percent of the samples did not have even 10 percent of the claimed number of live microorganisms.

For example, if a pure acidophilus was supposed to have 5 billion/g, it might not have even 500 million/g. More than 40 to 50 percent of the product could have more than one species. Several products even had microorganisms belonging to a genus other than lactobacillus; for example, in addition to *L. acidophilus*, they had *Lactococcus lactis*. Several of the samples even showed undesirable or pathogenic organisms present.

These are not only our observations; at least two papers in scientific journals authored by very renowned microbiologists have reported essentially similar results.[2, 3] Also, almost all acidophilus products carry promotional material with similar claims but without any literature identifying the research work and where it was published, or whether it was published in any peer-reviewed, reputable journal.

Some of the acidophilus products contain *Lactobacillus lactis* var. *rhamnosus* (or *L. rhamnosus*). Although *rhamnosus* has been reported to be a normal resident of the human gastrointestinal tract, little definitive scientific information is available concerning its nutritional importance. More recently a number of reports indicate that *L. rhamnosus* may very well be a good probiotic. Nevertheless, there does seem to exist considerable differences among various strains of *L. rhamnosus*.

*L. bulgaricus*, another food supplement on the market, and one of the two microorganisms used in the manufacture of yogurt (the other being *Streptococcus thermophilus*), is considered to be beneficial to the human organism. Significant research on *L. bulgaricus* has been done.

In order for any microorganism to continue to play any beneficial role beyond the period of time of its actual ingestion, it has to implant itself and multiply rapidly in the gut to avoid being expunged entirely.

The lactogenic bacteria must attach to the human intestinal cells, or mucosal cells. To achieve this, the bacteria must first be able to clinch to the mucosal surface. Second, our immune system must not reject the bacteria off the surface.[4]

For bacteria to successfully implant, the surface of the intestinal bacteria must be host-specific, in our case human-specific. Hence, if the culture is not human-specific, it may pass straight through the intestines and may not implant. These products are considered to be a waste of money.

Because DDS-1 was isolated from a human source, it is exceedingly well accepted by the human body, implanting and multiplying in the intestinal tract more easily than flora from animal strains, such as those used to make yogurt and some other flora supplements.

For gut inhabitation, *L. acidophilus* must not only be able to tolerate and pass through the high stomach acidity (low pH), but also be able to grow and proliferate at physiological levels of bile salts and adhere to the intestinal epithelial cells. Many bacteria are not tolerant to stomach acid and bile secretion in the small intestine.[5]

### Resiliency

The DDS-1 strain of acidophilus is incredibly resilient. Resiliency is crucial because it determines whether flora supplements are of any benefit at all. Many other strains of acidophilus are not resilient enough, and so do not ensure successful implantation in the intestinal tract. DDS-1 can survive in temperatures that kill many other strains and is resistant to moderate concentrations of bile salts. During the assimilation of foods, the gall bladder secretes bile salts into the intestine to break down, or emulsify, fats. These bile salts can also break down the fatty cell membranes of microbial cells, thus destroying the organisms. Sometimes this is good—in cases where harmful microorganisms enter the body through food—and sometimes this is unfortunate—in cases where flora supplements are being ingested.

*L. acidophilus* DDS-1 has been reported to be highly resistant to several commonly known antibiotics like penicillin, streptomycin, and aureomycin. Such antibiotic resistance of *L. acidophilus* DDS-1 is of paramount importance because it can be taken soon after an individual has been on antibiotic therapy, or even while currently taking antibiotics. Common antibiotic therapy not only kills the pathogenic bacteria but also kills "friendly bacteria" like lactobacilli and streptococci, and may upset gastrointestinal microbial balance. *L. acidophilus* DDS-1 can help in restoring the optimal microbial balance in the gut.

### Growth and Harvest

Bacterial cultures must be grown in the proper medium to ensure both abundant quantities and optimal biological activity. A liquid medium is used because only in this way can the solid material—the microorganisms—be isolated after growth. Because the solid and liquid substances have different densities and molecular sizes, they can be effectively separated by centrifugation, reverse osmosis, or ultrafiltration. The selection of the nutritional components of the medium is essential to ensure biological activity. In certain media, a particular species of microorganism will grow abundantly and be stable upon harvesting, while in other media, the same species will not achieve the same desirable characteristics. Because bacteria are alive, they require food to thrive. Probiotic companies have often added some type of "food" to their products, usually a carbohydrate such as a polysaccharide. The trend today is to include fructooligosaccharides (FOS) to support bacterial growth. This is an energy compound of specialty sugars that "drive" the bacteria and make them grow.[6]

### Manufacture of Freeze-Dried L. acidophilus DDS-1

For best results, *L. acidophilus* DDS-1 is manufactured by an exclusive process involving growth in a well-defined and highly nourishing medium for this special strain. In the manufacturing process, the microorganisms are concentrated first by removing unspent liquid medium by sedimentation, ultrafiltration, reverse osmosis, and/or centrifugation.

### Preservation

The technique used in the initial preservation of the flora is freeze-drying. Although freeze-drying is the least likely method to cause death to the microorganisms, cell damage is always a danger with extreme temperatures. A specific cryoprotectant is added to the intact cell concentrate before freezing to prevent "freezer damage" to the bacteria. More than ten cryoprotective agents researched and hand-picked by Dr. Shahani are added to his formulas to contribute additional stability to the cells. Some are amino acids, some are herbs, and some are antioxidants, such as vitamins C and E and glutathione, which can be utilized by the human body once ingested (antioxidants function to control the cell and tissue damage caused by free radicals, and thus contribute to the body's natural defenses). If flora are protected during freeze-drying, a majority of the cells are not killed, but are merely rendered dormant by the removal of necessary warmth and moisture. This dormant state means they will not multiply beyond the capacity of their container or capsule, and different strains will not compete with each other for space and food. Once inside the body, all essential life-giving factors are present, and so the flora will thus be reactivated.

Following freezing, the mass is freeze-dried in a specially designed unit. The final product is then subjected to fine screening and quality control involving over 30 rigorous quality-control tests. When the product passes all the rigorous tests, it is then mixed with a natural stabilizer to prevent the loss of its viability during packaging, shipping, storage, marketing, and consumption. Approved manufacturing is all done under the rigid controls stipulated by Dr. Shahani.

As far as is known, the viability of the cells is not damaged at all during sedimentation, ultrafiltration, reverse osmosis, or centrifugation, unless the processing equipment is faulty and/or the processor is not properly trained.

### Stability

*L. acidophilus* DDS-1 is highly stable even under adverse conditions of manufacture and storage. Normally, microorganisms such as *L. acidophilus* are affected adversely by heat, moisture or humidity, light, and air. The unique process of manufacturing DDS-1, coupled with the addition of a suitable cryoprotectant and specially designed natural stabilizers, protects the microorganisms against humidity (moisture), light, heat, and oxygen (from air), providing a stability unsurpassed as far as is known.[7]

Each factor in the production of these flora products is the result of many years of published research, special controls, and the influence of scientific experts and highly qualified and well-trained laboratory technicians.

## RESPONSIBILITES OF THE FOOD-SUPPLEMENT ADVOCATE

As indicated above, all of the different acidophilus products are *not* alike because they do not have similar properties or benefits. In addition, a known strain of *L. acidophilus*, even *L. acidophilus* DDS-1, manufactured by different methods, will not have similar properties and stability.

It is a serious concern that numerous food supplements on the market do not meet the standards claimed on their labels. The consumer has every right to demand that the product one purchases actually meets the standards or claims made for that product. It is therefore a serious responsibility of the health professional, and of the health food store as well, to make sure that the manufacturer and/or the supplier provides documented proof, preferably published in a peer-reviewed scientific journal or publication, that the claims made for the product were indeed substantiated by tests or research done with that product.

When someone makes a verbal claim on a product, ask what they base it on, and ask for written literature on that claim.

### Labeling Standards

As part of its ongoing quality-assurance effort, the NNFA Committee for Product and Label Integrity (ComPLI) has established a labeling standard for probiotic products. The standard requires probiotic supplement labels to provide the following:

- the quality and identity of living organisms present
- a suggested final date for use
- a statement of storage requirements
- a listing of additional ingredients.

## Delivery Mechanisms

Probiotic supplements are sold as liquids, powders, capsules, tablets, and chewable wafers. Each of these forms have unique attributes. Liquid products offer the least stability, mainly because the bacteria start growing when water and food are inherently available in a liquid. These new bacteria are fragile and they tend to die off.

Powders are sometimes more economical, but they may be more susceptible to moisture. Every time a bottle is opened during usage, particularly if it's in a refrigerator, condensation happens and moisture may get in.

One of the manufacturers of the DDS-1 strain, Nebraska Cultures, has developed a stabilizer that tends to offset the effects of heat, light, oxygen, and humidity. This does not mean that if you put it in a UPS truck and keep it in the heat, they will survive. The higher the temperature, the greater the loss. If acidophilus is left too long exposed to heat and humidity, the bacteria will start to regenerate or multiply, and they will consume the available food. When all the food is consumed, they will start dying off. That's why refrigeration is necessary. Any person or company telling you that *L. acidophilus* does not require refrigeration may be misinformed or misrepresenting their product.

Capsules, tablets, and chewable wafers offer ease of use. Capsules may offer additional protection from moisture provided by the surrounding capsule shell. Tablets are inherently not ideal because of processing conditions that may include heat, water, and compression, which would injure the bacterial cell walls, reducing their chances for regeneration. The manufacturing process for chewable wafers may be less damaging. Companies often compensate for this loss by starting the process with a much higher number of bacteria than the final label claim indicates.

When considering different probiotic products, the following points serve as a guide:

1. Buy human-specific bacteria. Of course, some strains of a specific culture have been shown to be interspecies-specific.

In other words, human-specific bacteria may implant in animals as well, and vice versa.

2. Make certain the bacterial strains used have proven to be stomach-acid and bile resistant and retain viability for several hours.

3. Always obtain an independent assay for viable counts.

4. Confirm that the probiotics are kept in cool storage from the point of manufacture through the point of distribution, up to the time they are shipped to you.

5. During warmer seasons, distributors should be shipping probiotics by overnight or 2-day service.

# Using Probiotics Throughout the Life Span

## Assessing Our Needs

### STOOL INDICATORS

For *L. acidophilus* and *B. bifidum* to be effective against the "bad guys," they must be present in extremely high numbers. In a stool culture, 50 percent to 100 percent of bowel bacteria such as lactobacillus is considered to be the healthy range.[1]

If you suspect that your digestive flora have been disrupted (typical symptoms include diarrhea, abdominal discomfort, and gas), and you want analytical testing confirmation, ask your physician to do a comprehensive stool analysis to check the proper balance of bacterial flora.

If the diagnosis is confirmed, you would be wise to add probiotics to your diet.

### PROBIOTIC THERAPY FOR ADULTS

Primarily, you'll need a probiotic supplement containing *L. acidophilus* that provides enough bacteria to recolonize your gut. Probiotics come in powder and capsule form, and in dairy-derived and dairy-free versions. We recommend that patients on antibiotic therapy start taking acidophilus probiotics while taking the antibiotics, and continue taking them for at least a month afterward.

The same advice goes to patients awaiting results of stool analysis. If the analysis indicates an imbalance, patients who take probiotics will have a head-start on the therapy, which can sometimes take up to 3 months to improve intestinal flora.

A daily dose of 15 to 20 billion organisms is required to combat acute infections.[2] An ideal maintenance dose is 3 to 7 billion organisms per day; this is suitable as a regular preventative dose for any healthy person. A high-quality acidophilus supplement will state on the package how many billion organisms are in each capsule or teaspoon.

## PROBIOTIC THERAPY FOR CHILDREN

A ratio of bifidobacteria and acidophilus is appropriate. We do know that the younger the child is, the more the formula should emphasize the bifidobacteria.[3]

There hasn't been much laboratory research on the actual needs of children. Based on clinical practice results, we find our recommendations for children are similar to that of adults, but in a lower dosage—1 to 2 billion ($1/4$ teaspoon of powder or one capsule) every day is adequate for the maintenance of a child's health. If there is a specific problem, 10 billion or one gram (2–3 capsules) is appropriate until the problem is resolved, then 1–2 billion is resumed.

## PROBIOTIC THERAPY FOR INFANTS

A blend emphasizing one-half *Bifidobacterium infantis, longum* and *bifidum,* and one-half *L. acidophilus* is best. Simply mix $1/4$ teaspoon (1–2 billion organisms) per day in juice, milk, or formula.

## Probiotics with Colostrum

In the first few days after birth and before the main milk flow, all female mammals (including humans) produce liquid colostrum. It is lower in fat and sugar (lactose) than milk and is much higher in protein. The colostrum protein is mostly immunoglobulins and antibodies. These antibodies protect the newborn from disease until its own immune system is working.

Besides protein, colostrum also contains hormones, enzymes, complex sugars, and a growth factor which speeds up tissue growth or tissue healing.

The greatest benefits provided by colostrum's immune factors are not in the blood or lymph, but actually inside the intestine and lung bronchii. Many people do not understand the use of colostrum, but it gets the bowel started right. It changes bowel activity for the better. People of all ages can benefit from taking colostrum. IgG is considered to be the most important immunoglobulin in the body. Of all the immunoglobulin in human milk, 2 percent is IgG, whereas IgG consititutes 86 percent of the immunoglobulin bovine colostrum. Bovine colostrum is accepted by virtually all mammals, including humans.

While fairly new in today's market, probiotic formulas with colostrum are expanding as more people realize its amazing unique benefits.

## Probiotic-Containing Foods

A logical question that arises is: Aren't there natural foods from which we can derive probiotics?

Definitely! There's a better concentration of lactobacilli in high-quality yogurts, buttermilk, sour cream, and kefir than in cow's milk or even mother's milk.

Fermented foods that have been cultured with microorganisms can include tempeh and other soy foods, miso, amazake, umeboshi plums, sour pickles, pickled vegetables, sauerkraut, sourdough bread, buttermilk, and yogurt. Even doctors worldwide have finally come to the conclusion that yogurt is a very beneficial product. Yogurt is typically made with two different bacteria: *Lactobacillus bulgaricus* and *Streptococcus thermophilus*.

However, yogurt and other foods can be fermented with many kinds of microorganisms, including lactobacillus; check the label to make sure you get what you think you're getting.

Vegetarians and people allergic to milk protein should note, however, that only dairy products contain significant levels of lactobacillus. If one cannot eat dairy foods, or chooses not to eat them, that person may take probiotic supplements instead. Even if you're healthy, taking supplements or eating foods fermented with *L. acidophilus* will help ensure that you have enough of these little helpers in your system. Indigenous peoples in the Middle East, India, and Asia have known about the therapeutic value of lactobacillus for thousands of years. They preserved foods and enhanced the foods' nutritional benefits by controlled fermentation of special cultures of bacteria. Now we know why these foods are so helpful.

# The Future

## *Prebiotics*

One of the most recent developments in the probiotic field, and one that has captured the attention of the probiotic researchers, has been the introduction of prebiotics. A prebiotic is defined as a "nondigestible food ingredient that beneficially affects the host by selectively stimulating the growth and/or activity of one or a limited number of bacteria in the colon, and thus improves host health." [Gibson, G. R., and M. B. Roberfroid. 1995. "Dietary modulation of the human colonic microbiota: introducing the concept of prebiotics," *J. Nutr.* 125:1401–12.] In other words, a prebiotic is a natural food material that is metabolized by only a select group of intestinal bacteria, whose growth is then stimulated at the expense of other microorganisms. To understand how prebiotics function, consider the analogy of a gardener tending to a lawn containing grass and weeds. A prebiotic would be like a special type of lawn food that supports growth of the grass, but not the weeds. The grass would grow and eventually displace the weeds. The same result would be achieved when prebiotics are ingested—the beneficial intestinal bacteria would grow and, over time, outcompete the undesirable bacteria, creating a healthier GI tract.

Similar to the case of probiotics, there are several criteria that must be satisfied for a food to be considered a prebiotic:

1. It must be neither hydrolyzed nor absorbed in the upper part of the gastrointestinal tract.
2. It must be selectively fermented by one or a limited number of potentially beneficial bacteria in the colon.
3. It must alter the composition of the colonic microbiota toward a healthier composition.
4. It must preferably induce effects that are beneficial to the host's health.

Among the foods and food ingredients that satisfy the above criteria, and that exhibit prebiotic activity, are a special class of carbohydrates called *oligosaccharides*. These exist naturally in many foods, including garlic, onions, bananas, chicory, milk, and soybeans. Several oligosaccharides, including fructooligosaccharides (FOS) and galactooligosaccharides (GOS), have been commercialized and are now used as ingredients in yogurt, cultured dairy products, and other foods, as well as in probiotic supplements. Although relatively few of these products are available in the United States, they are especially popular in Europe and Japan where more than 500 foods and nutritional supplements have been formulated with prebiotic oligosaccharides.

In theory, prebiotics consumed alone might be able to deliver beneficial effects, provided that the beneficial lactobacilli and bifidobacteria are indeed present in the GI tract in sufficient numbers. However, many of the probiotic supplements available in the marketplace now contain prebiotics. Such products (where probiotics and prebiotics are combined) are called *synbiotics*. This approach, therefore, may provide an efficient mechanism for introducing and then enriching health-promoting probiotic bacteria.

## Symbiosis and Total Health

*Symbiosis* is defined as "the intimate living of two kinds of organisms where the association is mutually advantageous."

Probiotics represent the ushering in of the future. The use of antibiotics will continue to play an important role in emergencies. Beyond this, the disease treatment and temporary "cure" approaches are becoming a concept of the past. The antibiotic detriments and side effects far too often outweigh their benefits.

Trends in the health field are emphasizing life-supportive antibiotic factors in daily lifestyles that focus on true correction and wholeness of well-being. This includes prevention, of course.

The type of diet you eat is a major influence on bacterial health. The bacteria are healthier on a diet rich in complex carbohydrates (vegetables, whole grains, legumes) and low in animal fats, fatty meat, sugars, and commercially processed dairy products. Experiments have found that common food additives like sodium benzoate and potassium sorbate actually kill good bacteria. Not surprisingly, the diet that is best for people is also ideal for healthy bacteria.

The fact is that microbes are a natural part of our existence. The realization that one can now selectively control the internal environment to one's advantage is a significant step forward in our understanding of health parameters. Nonetheless, a full understanding of the intimate relationship between "man and the microbe" is yet to unfold.

# Frequently Asked Questions

1. What is the importance of human gastrointestinal microflora?

   Inside each of us live vast numbers of bacteria (several trillion) that are necessary for good health. There are five major groups of bacteria that inhabit the human gut and many other minor groups. The five major groups include the bifidobacteria, lactobacilli, streptococci, bacteroides, and the coliforms. They all thrive in the warm, wet, and dark spaces inside animal bodies, and they compete vigorously to establish colonies. A healthy intestine is one that maintains a critical balance between the friendly and harmful bacteria. Any imbalance or the reduction of the friendly or beneficial bacteria results in ill health.

2. Why is it important to monitor these flora in the human gastrointestinal tract?

   If harmful bacteria grow too great in proportion, fairly serious consequences can result. Diseases such as rheumatoid arthritis, ankylosing spondylitis (rheumatoid arthritis of the spine), colitis, diabetes, meningitis, myasthenia gravis (a neuromuscular defect that causes muscular weakness and debility), thyroid disease, and bowel cancer are thought to have a connection with a significantly altered bowel flora. Substances produced by harmful bacteria have been shown to have tumor-promoting capabilities and to cause immune dysfunction and local inflammation.

3. When we hear the phrase "friendly flora," what are we talking about?

   We are talking about helpful bacteria rather than pathogenic (disease-causing) bacteria or germs. Among the five major bacteria in the gut, lactobacilli and bifidobacteria are considered to be beneficial and the coliforms are considered to be harmful bacteria. Many people aren't aware of it, but there is a predominance of friendly bacteria living in our intestines that actually work very hard to keep us from being infected by the pathogenic ones. So when a biologist talks about "friendly flora," that expert is talking about the populations of helpful microbes inhabiting the human gut.

4. Is it true that humans cannot digest food without the help of friendly flora?

Absolutely, and bacteria are a big help. When we eat, we first chew our food; enzymes are produced in the salivary gland that begin to break down that food. The chewed food is then subjected to strong hydrochloric acid in the stomach that further breaks it down. Finally, our bodies produce enzymes from the liver and pancreas to further help break down the particles. We do get a lot of digestive help from bacteria when the macro (large) particles are broken down into micro (small) particles by the action of enzymes produced by bacteria. Actually, the bacteria are digesting food for themselves and we indirectly benefit. In order to feed themselves, the bacteria produce their own enzymes that break macromolecules down into micromolecules—a size they can eat. We benefit from this because of their short and simple cycle of life. Bacteria reproduce and die off at an amazingly fast rate, and they leave residual enzymes for the host, which can be beneficial. An example of such a helpful enzyme would be lactase, which breaks down the lactose found in milk products.

5. Is it true that some people are lactose tolerant by nature and some are not?

I believe that nature produces whatever is necessary, and there is a strict economy in its production. People in Scandinavia, for example, have diets that feature abundant dairy products. In India the people have a lot of lactose in their diet in the form of cultured products like yogurt. These people tend to develop systems that produce adequate lactase as part of the economy of their natural processes. In Africa the diets do not contain an abundance of lactose, so it is not part of the metabolic system. In modern civilization, where pasteurization of milk products is the norm, we now see greater problems in the populations at large with their ability to metabolize dairy products or foods. The enzymes, which were inherent in the raw dairy products, are no longer present, leading to an entirely new health issue.

6. How do friendly flora help lactose-intolerant individuals?

Since lactase is one of the enzymes produced in large quantities by these friendly bacteria, it is conceivable that such a person could benefit from the lactase this friendly bacteria would produce in excess in his or her intestines.

7. What are the primary causes of microflora imbalance?

Travel is just one way to upset the balance of intestinal flora. Changing food habits, diets high in sugars, high heat-treated products, environmental contaminants, disrupted sleep cycles, and antimicrobial agents such as antibiotics can all affect our internal environments.

8. What damages the friendly bacteria, rendering them useless?

A high level of local acidity is one major detrimental influence. Acidity is created by certain types of diet, digestive function, and stress on the system. Another influence is the speed of peristalsis (the wavelike contraction of the intestines), which moves food along the digestive tract. If it is too rapid (as in diarrhea, irritable bowel syndrome, or colitis), this severely reduces the efficiency of the flora. If it is too slow (as in atonic or spastic constipation), this too causes changes in their function. The type of diet may have a major influence on bacteria health. The bacteria are healthier on a diet rich in complex carbohydrates (vegetables, whole grains, legumes) and low in animal fats and fatty meat. This diet, which is healthiest for people, is also ideal for the healthy bacteria. The friendly bacteria are also influenced to a major extent by the degree of infection by yeast and bacteria to which the bowel is subjected. Certain drugs, especially anti-biotics, can severely upset this delicate balance. Penicillin will kill friendly bacteria just as efficiently as it will kill disease-causing bacteria. Steroids (hormonal drugs) such as cortisone, ACTH, prednisone, and birth control pills also cause great damage to the healthy bowel flora.

9. Why are the friendly bacteria sometimes referred to as "lactic acid bacteria"?

The friendly bacteria produce lactic acid and are ofen re-ferred to as lactic acid bacteria. *Lactobacillus acidophilus* is one such example. Over millennia, humans have evolved a sym-biotic relationship with these bacteria. Although they are harmless to us, they have the ability to kill off other bacteria by secreting small quantities of antibioticlike substances, including lactic acid, acetic acid, benzoic acid, hydrogen peroxide, acidolin, lactocidin, and acidophilin. All these substances have a wide spectrum of activity against harmful, foodborne bacteria.

10. What is *Lactobacillus acidophilus?*

This is one of the friendly bacteria that consumes and metab-olizes sugars and produces lactic acid. It can be found in some fermented dairy products and nutritional supplements. When acidophilus is consumed in adequate numbers, it populates the intestinal tract and can enhance the state of health.

11. Acidophilus produces natural antibioticlike agents—are these agents potent?

Acidophilin, one of the antibioticlike substances produced by acidophilus, has more killing power than penicillin, strep-tomycin, or terramycin. Acidophilus is a virtual biochemical warrior with a devastating arsenal of weapons for wiping out disease-causing bacteria.

12. What is *Lactobacillus acidophilus* DDS-1?

It is a special strain of lactobacillus developed by the research group at the University of Nebraska. DDS-1 stands for Department of Dairy Science Strain No. 1.

13. What makes DDS-1 special?

The beneficial properties of this strain have been well documented over the years, something no other may claim. These healthful properties are based on research that has been documented in internationally reputable journals. Those documented benefits are as follows:

- Production of protease enzymes, which help us digest proteins, lactase for breaking down lactose, and lipase enzymes to help digest fats.
- Production of B vitamins, which are biocatalysts in food and metabolism, particularly folic acid and vitamin $B_{12}$.
- Production of acidophilin, which is a natural antibioticlike agent that inhibits 23 known toxic microorganisms.

Our research has demonstrated conclusively that there is a considerable difference between the different strains of lactobacillus. In fact, the very same strain grown under different conditions will show different properties. This is why DDS-1 is more than simply the particular strain of the species; it is a product of specific conditions of the culture and the processes. *L. acidophilus* DDS-1 is produced by a unique process that includes growing it in a special medium. It is then mixed with special *cryoprotective* (protecting against the cold) agents before it is freeze-dried. It is finally stabilized with a specially designed natural stabilizer to protect the microorganisms against moisture, light, heat, and humidity. This provides a stability that is unsurpassed to date. So, even this same strain of *L. acidophilus* DDS-1, if not produced by the University of Nebraska process, would not have the same beneficial properties and stability.

14. Is there an undesirable strain of *L. acidophilus* like the bad strain of *E. coli* found in tainted meat? Could one be harmed if one took heavy doses of *L. acidophilus*?

    In all my years of research, I have never encountered nor heard about any undesirable form of lactobacillus, like the undesirable species of streptococcus, which can cause strep throat.

15. What is *bifidus*?

    *Bifidobacterium bifidum* (previously known as *L. bifidus*) are beneficial intestinal bacteria that typically live in large numbers in the large intestine and colon. This differs from *Lactobacillus acidophilus*, which inhabits the small intestine. (*L. acidophilus* can be found in the colon, but it predominates in the small intestine). Bifidobacterium works synergistically with *L. acidophilus*. *L. acidophilus* and bifidobacterium are both necessary to maintain optimum health of the gastrointestinal tract. These can be combined to provide optimal health and protection for the digestive system.

16. What is *Enterococcus faecium?*

    *Enterococcus faecium* has been found to be an excellent food supplement; however, only certain strains of *E. faecium* have been found to have beneficial properties. Here, too, there are differences among the strains. The question has been raised whether *E. faecium* can be dangerous, whether it can cause migraine headaches, or produce histamines. The latest *Bergy Manual,* which is the "bible" for microbiologists, says specifically that *E. faecium* does not have an enzyme called decarboxylase, and any organism which does not have decarboxylase will not produce any amines from amino acids. Not only is *E. faecium* a safe product, it is an excellent product and is being used extensively in Europe. It has been adopted by the World Health Organization for use in Bangladesh where there is extensive incidence of diarrhea.

17. What are the natural foods from which we can derive acidophilus?

   Fermented foods like tempeh, miso, amazake, umeboshi plums, sour pickles, sauerkraut. However, be aware that yogurt and these other foods can be fermented with many kinds of microorganisms besides lactobacillus. In addition, many of these products are heat-treated after fermemtation, killing the bacteria. Most yogurts made in the United States contain acidophilus, but strain differences exist.

18. Which undesirable bacteria can the friendly flora control?

   Many studies have established conclusively the antibiotic effects of the friendly bacteria. In one study, 19 cases of nonspecific infections of the vagina were treated with acidophilus (Doderlein bacillus strain); 95 percent were cured. In another study of 25 cases of monila vaginitis, 88 percent were cured and 12 percent relieved of symptoms. In 444 cases of trichomonas vaginitis, 92 percent were cured and remained infection-free up to a year later. The antibioticlike agent acidophilin, which is produced by *L. acidophilus* DDS-1, has been shown to inhibit 27 different disease-causing bacteria. Sixteen children with salmonella poisoning and fifteen with shigella infections were cleared of all symptoms using acidophilus. *Bifidobacterium bifidum* effectively kills or controls *E. coli, Staphylococcus aureus* (the cause of toxic shock syndrome), and Shigella. Acidophilus can control viruses as well, such as herpes.

19. Can friendly flora prevent candidiacis?

   Observation shows that lactobacilli lack antifungal activity. However, it has been documented that *L. acidophilus* aids in the production or augmentation of immune bodies and functions, and these may inhibit candida (yeast) infection.

20. How can we diagnose the presence and type of pathogenic microbes, the degree of intestinal damage, and/or the extent of compromised immunity? How can one know if antibiotics or other factors have disrupted the digestive flora?

Any gastrointestinal disorders, such as gas, flatulence, pain, diarrhea and dysentery, or bloody stool may indicate the presence of pathogenic organisms in the intestine. By culturing stool samples, one may detect or determine the kinds of pathogenic organisms. Persistence of unhealthy gastrointestinal disorders may also reflect compromised immunity.

21. Since diarrhea is a common symptom that is directly related to an imbalance of intestinal flora, will you comment on some of the strains of bacterial species capable of causing this miserable condition?

In the United States we view diarrhea as an inconvenient misery, but in other parts of the world diarrhea is a killer. This is especially true of children, where more than half a million under the age of 5 die each year due to uncontrollable diarrhea: dysentery, caused by Shigella or cholera, caused by *Vibrio cholera*—incidentally, both are species of coliform. Some organisms may produce diarrhea without establishing a colony in the intestines. *Staphylococcus aureus*, some strains of clostridium, typhoid, and *Bacillus cereus* produce and release toxins in food and in the human intestines that can cause diarrhea. On the other hand, *Escherichia coli*, Salmonella, Shigella, and Vibrio must colonize the intestine where their proliferation determines the course of the disease.

22. Harmful bacteria will produce toxins that make the host sick. How does that work?

Mainly, they produce enzymes that catalyze reactions that don't do us any good. For example, histidine decarboxylase is an enzyme that alters the amino acid histidine to histamine, and histamine can cause headaches. Also, tyrosine can be catalyzed to tyramine, which is the substance providing the odor of decaying dead bodies.

23. What is intestinal toxemia and how can it be eliminated?

Intestinal toxemia refers to the fact that we can literally poison our own systems by way of our intestinal tract. If we eat the wrong kinds and amounts of food, bacteria in the intestine will feed on these improper food items and produce toxins that will be absorbed into the bloodstream. There are three basic requirements for eliminating intestinal toxemia:

(1) Cleansing the system of long-term accumulated toxins. There are various approaches offered today, some mild, some intense. Numerous approaches can be beneficial. This can be determined on an individual basis by a qualified health professional.

(2) Dietary lifestyle improvements. Cutting out refined sugars, refined flour, and some other dietary products can improve elimination. Beyond this, there may be dietary changes that must be made that are unique for each individual situation and health condition. This must be determined on an individual basis by a qualified health professional.

(3) Replenish the system adequately with proper quantities of a high-quality probiotic flora. To truly conquer this problem and attain lasting health, all three of these steps are critical for most people today.

24. What is meant by probiotics?

Certain bacteria help to maintain good health and certain bacteria have a definite value in helping us regain health once it has been upset. These dual protective and therapeutic roles of certain bacteria explain why the word "probiotics" was coined. Probiotics means "for life." Probiotics have been defined as organisms, such as friendly bacteria, which contribute a great deal to the health and balance of the intestinal tract, thus benefiting us by protecting against disease and improving nutrition. They are live microorganisms that can enhance our state of health.

25. What do probiotics do?

Probiotics contribute to our digestion and nutrition, reduce cholesterol levels, counteract the negative effects from antibiotic therapy, and improve our immune system.

26. How do probiotics contribute to our digestion and nutrition?

Here, the probiotics contribute in many ways:
- They enhance the digestion and absorption of protein.
- They improve the digestion and absorption of fat.
- They may increase the absorption and retention of minerals such as phosphorus, calcium, and iron.
- They may lessen the severity of allergic response to milk.
- They produce some B vitamins and possibly vitamin K.

27. How do probiotics contribute to cholesterol reduction?

Some preliminary research has produced promising results in lowering serum cholesterol with the dietary use of lactobacilli. Future research will indicate how many bacteria are needed for a beneficial effect.

28. How do probiotics counteract the negative effects of antibiotic therapy?

Individuals who have undergone antibiotic therapy frequently report a normalization of intestinal function when they take probiotic preparations.

29. How do probiotics contribute to our immune system?

It has been documented that lactobacilli may enhance white blood cell activity (specifically the macrophage cells and lymphocytes). This means that the immune system becomes more powerful and more effective. Lactobacilli produce lactic acid in the gastrointestinal tract and this helps prevent the growth of harmful bacteria (pathogens). Lactobacilli produce natural nontoxic, antibioticlike agents that can inhibit the growth of some pathogenic bacteria in the gastrointestinal tract. When the lactobacilli have successfully colonized the gastrointestinal tract, they may prevent the growth of harmful microorganisms like *Candida albicans* and *Clostridia.*

30. Who needs probiotics or might benefit from their use? Do most people need probiotic supplementation?

Individuals who would benefit from probiotics are those who take antibiotics, some cortisonelike drugs, birth control pills, alcohol, some food additives, caffeine, chlorinated or fluoridated water, and processed foods, as well as those on high-fat and high-sugar diets which can destroy the natural intestinal flora. Ideally, we should completely avoid factors that can disturb our bacterial ecosystem. For most people this is impossible. Probiotic supplementation, then, is a vital way to promote good health. These supplements can help offset the disturbing effect that dietary, environmental, and emotional stresses create in the GI tract.

Since it has been established that we all need 3–4 pounds of healthy intestinal flora, anyone who may have disrupted this balance could benefit from probiotics. The disruption could have occurred due to various lifestyle factors, especially the utilization of antibiotics (which are also in much of the meat we eat today). Even if you are healthy, taking probiotic supplements or eating foods fermented with *L. acidophilus* will help ensure that you have enough of the little critters in your system. People of the Middle East, India, and Asia have known about the therapeutic value of lactobacillus for thousands of years. They preserved foods and enhanced the foods' nutritional benefits by controlled fermentation of special cultures of bacteria.

31. What are some of the factors that help probiotics to grow?

    Probiotics are, in fact, a lot like us. They grow on good quality food, they grow on water, and they grow on what we call love and affection.

32. What are full-spectrum probiotics and how do they perform?

    Full-spectrum probiotics refers to products containing *L. acidophilus*, bifidobacteria, and usually one to eight additional good bacterial species. These full-spectrum formulas may be considered to do a better job than the acidophilus and bifidum alone. These products may have an edge over the single strains. They will also assist those individuals who may have a tendency toward diarrhea symptoms and other gastrointestinal disorders.

33. Can we effectively combine a full spectrum of beneficial bacteria? Is there scientific validity to the rumor of "cannibalism" among the microorganisms? Is it desirable or advantageous to take a mixture of microbial food supplements, containing such organisms as *L. acidophilus* and *B. bifidum*, or any other probiotic organisms? There has been much debate about whether different microorganisms present in a mixed microbial supplement compete with or kill each other.

    Although it is a widely believed myth that probiotics should not be taken together, the rumors of "cannibalism" among the microorganisms are not scientifically valid. On the contrary, a healthy bacterial population includes many types of flora cohabiting peacefully. They do not fight with each other—the more the merrier. However, actively growing bacteria can inhibit each other. It is what they call "survival of the fittest." This is their biological phenomenon while growing. But, in supplements, most of these bacteria are in dry-powder or freeze-dried form. Probiotics in the freeze-dried form are in "suspended animation" and they do not begin multiplying until they are in a suitable environment. Once they start growing, they behave complementarily to one another. A two- or three-microorganism combination, if selected properly, can provide supplementary and complementary effects and thereby provide better benefits to the consumer. Each microorganism will seek its own best environment, whether that's the small intestine for *L. acidophilus*, the colon for *B. bifidum*, or the upper GI tract for *L. salivarius*; they are not likely to adversely affect the other species.

34. When is the best time to take acidophilus or other microbial supplements? Can they be taken on an empty stomach?

   I have said time and again that it is not advisable to take probiotics on an empty stomach. Probiotics need food, water, and warmth to flourish and multiply. All living systems need these three things. When you wake up each day, there is water in the body, the body is warm, and there is some food, but not enough for the probiotics to grow. When you provide your body with good food each day, you also nourish the probiotics. Take any probiotics along with a meal, just before or just after the meal.

35. Does the stomach acidity destroy the probiotic if it is taken with a meal?

   It will be destroyed to a certain extent, but it is negligible. A meal or its components may also act as a buffering system to the acidophilus. It is very important to take the probiotic with a meal so that the microorganisms can be nourished and grow. When taken with food, this helps avoid excessive exposure of the probiotic to the acid environment of an empty stomach.

36. When should one start or stop taking probiotics? How long can it take to improve an imbalance of intestinal flora?

   Beyond correction of a depleted system, probiotics are important on a maintenance/prevention basis. They are used to counteract any deficiency in the body that may occur because of lifestyle habits, ill health, and/or gastrointestinal problems. Not taking them is like not taking your food. Because probiotics maintain a healthy balance in the system, they can be likened to an insurance policy that protects physical belongings in the case of theft, fire, or some other catastrophe.

37. What are the symptoms for probiotic depletion and/or is there such a thing as a clinical indication for any probiotic product?

The friendly bacteria naturally promote bulky, well-lubricated stools and normal frequency of bowel movements, and they help counteract harmful bacteria. Most people usually have a moderate population of this friendly flora and take their activity for granted. But when depletion takes place, there is such a thing as clinical indication, consisting of persistence of diarrhea and/or constipation, and/or infrequent infections. The distress of small, hard, difficult-to-pass or infrequent stools may occur, as well as effects caused by toxins due to overgrowth of the harmful bacteria.

38. After implementing a course of probiotics and improving dietary factors, what signs of success should one expect?

In order for *L. acidophilus* and *B. bifidum* to be effective, they must be present in extremely high quantities. In a stool culture, 50 to 100 percent of bowel bacteria, such as lactobacillus, is considered to be the healthy range. Of course, other signs of success include diminished adverse symptoms and a greater sense of health and well-being.

39. What daily dose is required to combat acute infection?

A daily dose of 1 billion to 10 or 15 billion organisms may constitute a good dose, depending upon the severity of the situation.

40. Is antibiotic use ever warranted and, if so, when and how does one know when it is appropriate?

The use of antibiotics is warranted in serious infection when analysis of a culture indicates the pathogrens would be killed by antibiotics, and it is determined that the patient has no sensitivity to the antibiotics. But their use should be limited to the fullest possible extent, avoiding, in particular, the broad-spectrum drugs that destroy the Gram-negative intestinal and vaginal "good guy" bacteria. Also, viral illnesses are often still inappropriately treated with antibiotics. A great reduction in the use of these drugs would result from careful differentiation of these "viral" infections from the "bacteria" infections. So-called antibiotics do not work on the viruses.

41. What probiotics would you recommend for someone with systemic candida and how much/how often/how long should they be taken?

In general, probiotics do not have a direct inhibiting effect on candida, but probiotics enhance or augment the immune system of the individual and thereby may be able to affect candida. We are in the process of working out additional formulations that will be especially designed for candida. I cannot make any recommendations at this time, and I do not know whether anyone can. Probiotics do enhance the immune factors and our products do better than most; therefore, they may have some effect against candida. By establishing and maintaining higher levels of the normal microbial populations of the GI tract, less desirable organisms should not flourish as easily.

42. How about little babies, infants—do they need lactobacilli?

Nature takes the best care of that. When we are born, our intestinal tracts have no microbes in them at all. Newborn infants are inoculated with bacteria from their mother's milk. In the early days of microbiology, scientists thought that the observed "Gram-positive" bacteria were lactobacilli, but these have since been reclassified as bifidobacteria. Interestingly, researchers have found that there is both a quality and a quantity difference in "friendly flora" between infants who are nursed by their mothers and infants fed bottle formula. Those babies who are exclusively breast fed have far fewer bouts of diarrhea and cholic than do bottle-fed infants. We also know that the bifidobacteria are responsible for the reduced frequency of diarrhea in breast-fed infants.

43. Can probiotic flora formulas be used as a vaginal douche for vaginal and/or bladder infections and how?

Yes, use 4 capsules or 1–2 teaspoons of powdered acidophilus. Empty the powder into 2 ounces of warm water. Use this as a douche 1 to 2 times daily (depending upon the severity) until the condition has been resolved.

44. Which microbial food supplements are commonly used and why?

Only those supplements which possess nutritional and beneficial properties should be used. They include *Lactobacillus acidophilus*, *L. bifidus*, *L. bulgaricus*, *E. faecium*, and others. Research has demonstrated that only some special strains of each of the genus or species of bacteria are beneficial.

45. Are microorganisms on the GRAS list, and can you elaborate on the GRAS list?

GRAS stands for "Generally Recognized As Safe." Foods like bread, lettuce, and milk are not necessarily on the GRAS list. Foods from our general consumption patterns are traditionally considered safe even if they are not on the GRAS list. Similarly, some of the bacteria that are used in the manufacture of certain fermented foods or microbial supplements are considered automatically safe. Certain bacteria may be found on the GRAS list, but bacteria like *Lactococcus lactis, E. faecium, L. acidophilus, L. bifidus, L. bulgaricus, L. thermophilus* are not on the GRAS list, yet are generally recognized as safe.

46. Is there such a thing as a truly nondairy acidophilus or microbial supplement?

   Yes, with the updated knowledge of biotechnology, micro-organisms can and have been modified to grow with all the beneficial properties in a specially designed milk-free medium. Only experienced researchers and specialists, however, know these procedures.

47. I have heard that research has identified strains grown on milk sources as producing the most powerful probiotics?

   That's not really true. What the strain is grown on is only one part of the process. What the strain is originally isolated from is what's especially important. The strongest strains have been isolated from milk sources. That is true for many of the bacteria—not all of them. After you isolate the organism you can grow it on any number of nutrient media. Preferred media include soybeans, mung beans, and garbonzo beans. The strongest strains developed yet at the University of Nebraska—which probably has one of the most active lactic-acid-culture research projects in the world—were grown on garbonzo beans and other media.

48. What is involved in maintaining a healthy population of probiotic flora in one's intestinal tract?

   It is not enough for the probiotics to simply be present in the body. It is necessary that they implant themselves. This means that they must adhere to and colonize the intestinal wall. When this occurs maximally, the "bad bacteria" have no place to implant and are thus inhibited. Until the friendly flora dominate the intestinal mucosal wall, the bad guys will exist there. Even if one is taking probiotics consistently, if implantation does not occur, the bad guys may continue their territorial hold.

49. Is implantation difficult to achieve?

When a good probiotic is taken, some beneficial results are obtained, but this may stop when the supplementation stops because the probiotics have not implanted sufficiently. Without proper nourishment, they often pass right through. It may take several months or even longer before effective implantation is obtained. By ingesting the probiotic with meals and further enhancing this with the addition of enzymes, the consumer more likely obtains the adequate nourishment he or she needs. With a healthy, assimilated diet, these probiotics grow and multiply and a good implantation can often be achieved within weeks. Then by continuing a good diet and adequate dosages of probiotics, the implanted probiotics grow, multiply, and persist.

50. How long does it take to obtain successful implantation?

I recommend that patients on antibiotic therapy start taking acidophilus supplements while taking the antibiotics, continuing for at least a month afterward at therapeutic levels, and then going on to maintenance doses. I give the same advice to patients awaiting the results of stool analysis. If the analysis indicates an imbalance, patients will have a jump on the therapy; it can take weeks and sometimes up to 3 months to improve intestinal flora.

51. Does *L. acidophilus* need to be of human origin to be effective, and do we need to do an enema for 2–3 days with good quality whey to acidify the colon and then use a lactobacillus implant for it to be effective?

*L. acidophilus* does not have to be of human origin. Many acidophilus strains are interspecies-implantable. Human-origin acidophilus is isolated from fecal matter, which could be infected with viruses as well. It is better to have a strain that has been proven undoubtedly to be implantable—such as DDS-1.

There are many views regarding the appropriate method of giving a lactobacillus implant. Most people do not require acidification of the colon prior to implant. There may be certain cases where this will be required, but not normally. The stabilization system we use involves glycine and glutathione. These enhance the possibility of implantation because they enhance the permeability of the mucus membrane in the intestinal tract.

52. Are all *L. acidophilus* strains or cultures the same?

No. The *L. acidophilus* called DDS-1 is a unique strain that was developed by the author (Dr. Khem Shahani) at the University of Nebraska. The other flora strains that we use are also proprietary; but certain processing steps involve a proprietary stabilization process and the use of some micronutrients, such as vitamins and minerals.

53. Is there any data that substantiates that the flora products do indeed pass through the stomach, surviving the stomach acid and bile, and successfully implant in the intestines?

Yes, there are references on the gastric survival of probiotics. I know of at least eight that definitely substantiate their successful transit.

54. How can one be sure that a product is reliable?

You have to depend on your supplier. This places a very serious responsibility on the supplier. The supplier must be able to clarify to the consumer that the product does contain the organisms that are mentioned on the label, that the product contains the correct count, and that they are all stable over a period of time; the supplier must have done research on its own products to show this. These are all very important factors.

55. How are the products tested for purity, toxicity, elemental makeup, and potency?

It is essential that very stringent quality-control procedures be applied to identify heavy metal contaminants and anything unusual in the products that is of microbiological, physical, or chemical origin. Also, enumeration of the viable counts must be made, using standard, well-established, microbiological methods. The results should be published in reputable journals or books.

56. Is it very simple to test for microbial counts and strain identification, and are all laboratories qualified to do so?

The National Nutritional Foods Association (NNFA) has been on the bandwagon for some time to establish requirements for standardized testing procedures for enumeration and speciation (determining the strain by DNA analysis). All good analytical laboratories should be able to test for microbial counts (enumeration). However, speciation is a more complex and expensive process, and there are fewer laboratories in the country that can do speciation of microorganisms.

57. Can friendly bacteria be damaged during manufacture?

This depends on whether the manufacturer has done enough research work to establish and standardize optimal conditions of fermentation, freezing, and freeze-drying to produce a viable and stable product.

58. What does stabilized flora mean?

It means that the probiotic flora has been created in such a way that it is strong and stable enough to survive and make it past the acids of the stomach and/or be stable or retain viability during storage and shipping.

59. How are microbial supplements manufactured and stabilized?

To provide a superior supplement, bacteria with beneficial and therapeutic properties must be selected. There are hundreds of different strains of *Lactobacillus acidophilus*. All do not possess the same beneficial properties. After the proper type of bacterium is selected, one has to select the right medium in which to grow the bacteria. The choice is critical and usually only known to researchers. After the bacteria are grown, they are removed from the medium, which is called harvesting or concentration. After concentration, cryoprotective agents are added to the mixture and it is freeze dried. After freeze-drying and blending, another stabilizer is added for storage purposes.

60. What is the best manufacturing process for probiotics?

Presently, we incorporate the best scientific methods known when we manufacture DDS-1 acidophilus. A description of this manufacturing process is the best way to illustrate this.

At Nebraska Cultures, Inc., *L. acidophilus* DDS-1 is manufactured by an exclusive, unique process involving growth in a well-defined and highly nourishing medium for this special strain. In the manufacturing process, the microorganisms are first concentrated by removing unspent liquid medium by sedimentation, ultrafiltration, reverse osmosis, and/or centrifugation. The viability of the cells is not damaged during these processes unless the processing equipment is faulty and/or the processor is not properly trained. There is no convincing research data establishing that centrifugation is harmful to bacteria. Following freezing, the mass is freeze dried in a specially designed unit. The final product is then subjected to fine screening and quality control that involves more than ten rigorous tests. When the product passes all the tests, it is then mixed with a natural stabilizer to prevent the loss of its viability during packaging, shipping, storage, marketing, and consumption.

61. When *Lactobacillus acidophilus* is cultured commercially, as it is with DDS-1, it is a living organism that must be somehow encapsulated and packaged so that it reaches the consumer still in good enough condition to be effective as a supplement. How can this be done? What is the best way to store DDS-1 capsules?

Once we have established a viable culture, the bacteria remain alive for a very long time, as long as they are held at a very cold temperature. They can be frozen and held at 20° F—a suspended animation temperature, if you will—and the bacteria are not damaged. They can leave the freezer to be transported and refrozen without serious damage as long as they are not kept in warm temperatures for long periods of time. When they are ingested and warmed up to body temperature, they become filled with life and go to work. A frozen culture or bottle of capsules with the proper culture of DDS-1 will retain billions of viable bacteria for a long time at very low temperatures.

The notion that freezing the capsules, then removing the bottle from the freezer daily, will somehow create a harmful moisture problem is *not* true. The only thing that can be hurt by moving the bottle in and out of the freezer to take daily supplementation is the label on the bottle.

62. Has testing been done on the viability of probiotics when shipping them during hot summer months. If so, what are the results? In California, from June to September, temperatures in UPS trucks may be above 120° F for periods of time. Can probiotics be shipped in hot weather without any more loss of viability than would occur at temperatures below 75° F?

Heat, light, oxygen, and humidity can all damage the probiotic products. There are special stabilizers in DDS-1 products to maintain their integrity. However, it is best to have them shipped overnight or by second–day air and to keep them in a dark, cool place. These products are stable for 3 to 6 months at 55–60° F, unless they are abused (subjected to heat, light, oxygen, and humidity).

63. It would simplify things immensely if we could just eliminate the necessity for keeping acidophilus in the refrigerator. There are a goodly number of acidophilus products (and multiple-strain products) that have gone through the complete freeze-drying process and do not seem to require refrigeration. Could you comment on this?

We have not encountered any probiotic on the market that does not require refrigeration. Our survey has shown that 90 percent of the products on the market contain much lower viable counts than are claimed on the label—presumably because the viability was lost during shipping and storage (assuming the count was correct when the product was packaged).

Our products, in general, provide at least a 20–30 percent higher count than is indicated on the bottle. Our products are much more resistant to heat, light, oxygen, and humidity. Of course, the higher the temperature, the greater the chance of product loss. After a bottle is opened, it is exposed to humidity, oxygen, and light.

You will get better value and results if you put the lid on tightly and keep the bottle in the refrigerator. If it is consumed quickly, for example within 10–15 days, it can be kept at room temperature. Because of the fast consumption, there will still be enough probiotic to give you what you need. If kept at room temperature for this short period of time, the loss is negligible. Our research has shown that when our products are kept in the refrigerator for up to 2 years, they still tested high in potency. The product will reflect minimal loss of viable, active bacteria and will retain its active bacterial potency as long as the product is not abused with excessive exposure to heat, light, oxygen, or humidity.

64. Does emptying out the capsules and dissolving the contents in water compromise effectiveness of a probiotic product. Many vegetarians prefer to do this?

The probiotic should retain its efficacy whether taken out of the capsule or not. In general, however, vegetarians may prefer to purchase a product in all-vegetable capsules, as opposed to standard gelatin capsules.

65. What is the best form in which to purchase microorganisms—powder-capsule or tablet?

There is no fundamental difference—it depends on the preference of the consumer. The powder form provides the highest viable count, is the purest and most effective, and offers the most value for its cost. Capsules are a little more expensive because of the cost of the encapsulating process, but are considered more convenient than powder.

66. Why do some people put enzymes in the flora product? What is the advantage of that?

The enzymes are there to digest the nutrients—to feed the flora more effectively. They are just working on the food itself. Realize that all enzymes are highly substrate-specific. The enzymes in these probiotic formulas are specific for protein, fat, and carbohydrates. The enzymes don't digest anything in the capsule because the moisture content is too low to activate the enzyme. Below about 8 percent moisture, enzymes will be totally inactive. So, until these capsules enter our GI tract, no enzyme activity is occurring. Combining enzymes with probiotics is logical since both aid digestion.

67. Does the addition of enzymes to flora products digest and deactivate the flora? Can enzymes like protease harm the probiotic bacteria?

No. Food-based enzymes, like protease, do not harm or inhibit bacteria, particularly in a dry or freeze-dried condition.

In fact, bacteria are living microorganisms and when they multiply they produce their own enzymes. However, after a bacterium is dead, enzymes can then digest the bacteria.

68. What is meant by FOS?

   FOS stands for fructooligosaccharide. It is a naturally occurring carbohydrate that doesn't do anything to the bacteria in the capsule. Theoretically, this carbohydrate passes through the GI tract, and once it reaches the lower intestine, it is supposed to help nourish the beneficial bacteria naturally residing there, helping them to reproduce. This is a relatively new concept that still requires further development and research to determine all its scientific ramifications.

69. Can powdered acidophilus be taken with any liquid?

   Yes, you can use any juice or put it on anything you want. It can be taken with food, and has been shown to be more effective this way. It is still useful to take it without food, but it is more effective with food.

70. Which is the better material in which to bottle a probiotic product, glass or plastic?

   As far as can be ascertained, there is no documented research report available in the literature that has established, unequivocally, the superiority of one type of bottle over the other. The four elements most destructive to probiotic potency are heat, humidity, light, and oxygen. No one has proved by scientifically controlled experiments that glass prevents the transmission of any of those four elements more efficiently than plastic. I have always recommended the use of white plastic bottles on the basis of the fact that glass bottles are more liable to break in transit and are heavier, thereby costing more to ship. Another potential disadvantage of the amber-colored bottle is that it may have a tendency to absorb and retain more heat. Also, we believe that a white bottle possesses the aesthetic value associated with being regarded as clean and pure.

71. What is the normal storage and shelf life of probiotics?

There is no exact standard: the length varies with the individual strains and the manufacturing process and storage conditions.

72. When are the University of Nebraska probiotics with the new patent going to be available?

They are available now. *L. acidophilus* DDS-1, manufactured by the special proprietary process of Nebraska Cultures, Inc., and stabilized by a unique stabilizer, has been available for some time.

73. Is there a comprehensive book on probiotics that you could recommend?

Until now, there has been no reliable, comprehensive, scientifically authoritative book on the subject. We have combined our research into this book format to meet the interested and educated consumer's demands. However, one can also get a good amount of information from proceedings of numerous probiotic-related conferences and meetings that may be open to the public.

# References

## Introduction to the Gastrointestinal System

1. *Webster's New World Dictionary*, 2nd college edition. Simon and Schuster, New York, 1984.

2. *Longman Dictionary of Contemporary English*. Longman Publishers, UK, 1987.

3. Guyton, A. C. *Textbook of Medical Physiology*, 6th edition. W. B. Saunders Company, 1981, p. 560.

## Antibiotics

1. *Longman Dictionary of Contemporary English*. Longman Publishers, UK, 1987.

2. Levy, S. B. 1988. The challenge of antibiotic resistance. *Sci. Am.* 278(3):47–53.

3. Gaskin, I. M. *Spiritual Midwifery*, 4th edition. Book Publishing Company, 2000.

4. Tanner, J. T. 1999. The antibiotic dilemma: Emerging antibiotic resistance. *Food Testing and Analysis*, pp. 7, 8, 28.

5. Op den Camp, H. J. M., A. Obsterhof, and J. H. Veerkamp. 1985. Interaction of bifidobacterial lipoteichoic acid with human intestinal epithelial cells. *Infect. Immun.* 47:332–34.

6. Yanabe, M., M. Shibuya, T. Gonda, H. Asai, T. Tanaka, T. Narita, K. Sudo, and K. Itoh. 1999. Establishment of specific pathogen-free rabbit colonies with limited-flora rabbits associated with conventional rabbit flora, and monitoring of their cecal flora. *Exp. Anim.* 48(2):101–6.

7. Myles. *Textbook for Midwives*, 12th edition. Churchill Livingstone, September 1993.

8. Stewart, D. *The Five Standards of Safe Childbearing.* Napsac Reproductions, June 1981.

9. Levy, S. B. 1988. The challenge of antibiotic resistance. *Sci. Am.* 278(3):47–53.

## Homeostasis

1. *Webster's New World Dictionary*, 2nd college edition. Simon and Schuster, New York, 1984.

2. *Longman Dictionary of Contemporary English*. Longman Publishers, UK, 1987.

3. Guyton, A. C. *Textbook of Medical Physiology*, 6th edition. W. B. Saunders Company, 1981, p. 560.

4. Gaskin, I. M. *Spiritual Midwifery*, 4th edition. Book Publishing Company, 2000.

5. Myles. *Textbook for Midwives*, 12th edition. Churchill Livingstone, September 1993.

6. Stewart, D. *The Five Standards of Safe Childbearing.* Napsac Reproductions, June 1981.

7. Myles. *Textbook for Midwives*, 12th edition. Churchill Livingstone, September 1993.

8. Op den Camp, H. J. M., A. Obsterhof, and J. H. Veerkamp. 1985. Interaction of bifidobacterial lipoteichoic acid with human intestinal epithelial cells. *Infect. Immun.* 47:332–34.

9. Yanabe, M., M. Shibuya, T. Gonda, H. Asai, T. Tanaka, T. Narita, K. Sudo, and K. Itoh. 1999. Establishment of specific pathogen-free rabbit colonies with limited-flora rabbits associated with conventional rabbit flora, and monitoring of their cecal flora. *Exp. Anim.* 48(2):101–6.

10. Nakagawa, R., H. Hirakawa, T. Iida, T. Matsueda, and J. Nagayama. 1999. Maternal body burden of organochlorine pesticides and dioxins. *J. AOAC Int.* 82(3):716–24.

11. Levy, S. B. 1988. The challenge of antibiotic resistance. *Sci. Am.* 278(3):47–53.

12. Judith DeCava. Adjunctive tips. *Candiphobia*, vol. 3, no. 1.

13. Benzmark, S. 1998. Ecological control of the gastrointestinal tract. The role of probiotic flora. *Gut* 42:2–7.

## Introducing the Probiotics

1. *Webster's New World Dictionary*, 2nd college edition. Simon and Schuster, New York, 1984.

2. *Longman Dictionary of Contemporary English.* Longman Publishers, UK, 1987.

3. Shahani, K. M. and A. D. Ayebo. 1980. Role of dietary lactobacilli in gastrointestinal microecology. Proc. VI International Symposium on Intestinal Microecology. *Am. J. of Clin. Nutr.* 33(11):2448–57.

4. Fernandez, C. F., K. M. Shahani, and M. A. Amer. 1988. Control of diarrhea by lactobacilli. *J. of App. Nutr.* 40(1):32–42.

5. Friend, B. A. and K. M. Shahani. 1984. Nutritional and therapeutic aspects of lactobacilli. *J. of App. Nutr.* 36:126–36.

6. Petersdorf, R. G. *Principles of Internal Medicine.* McGraw Hill, New York, 1983, pp. 359–60.

7. Benzmark, S. 1998. Ecological control of the gastrointestinal tract. The role of probiotic flora. *Gut* 42:2–7.

8. Mitsuoka, T. 1984. The effect of nutrition on intestinal flora. *Nahrung* 28:619–25.

## Probiotics and Human Nutrition

1. Friend, B. A. and K. M. Shahani. Fermented Dairy Products, in *Comprehensive Biotechnology*, vol. 3 (C. L. Cooney and A. E. Humphrey, eds). Pergmon Press, New York, 1985, pp. 567–92.

2. Metchnikoff, Elie. *The Prolongation of Life* (P. Chalmer Mitchell, ed.). G. P. Putnam's Sons, The Knickerbocker Press, New York and London, 1908.

3. Wingrove, J., A. J. Bond, A. J. Cleare, and R. Sherwood. 1999. Plasma tryptophan and trait aggression. *J. Psychopharmacology*, 13:235–37.

4. Shahani, K. M. and K. C. Chandan. 1979. Nutritional and healthful aspects of cultured and culture-containing dairy foods. *J. of Dairy Sci.* 62:1685–94.

5. Ayebo, A. D., I. A. Angelo, and K. M. Shahani. 1981. Effect of ingesting *Lactobacillus acidophilus* milk upon fecal flora and enzyme activity in humans. *Milchwissenschaft* 35:730–33.

6. Shahani, K. M. and B. A. Friend. 1983. Properties of and prospects for cultured dairy products, in *Food Microbiology* (F. A. Skinner and T. A. Roberts, eds.). Academic Press, Inc.; London; pp. 257–69.

7. Butler, C. and J. W. Beakley. 1960. Bacterial flora in vaginitis. *Am. J. Obstet. Gynecol.* 7:432.

8. Lee, H., B. A. Friend, and K. M. Shahani. 1988. Factors affecting the protein quality of yogurt and acidophilus milk. *J. Dairy Sci.* 71:3222–28.

9. Fernandes, C. F. and K. M. Shahani. 1989. Lactose intolerance and its modulation with lactobacilli and other microbial supplements. *J. of App. Nutr.* 41:50–64.

10. Peuhkuri, K., M. Hukkanen, R. Beale, J. M. Polak, H. Vapaatalo, and R. Korpela. 1997. Age and continuous lactose challenge modify lactase protein expression and enzyme activity in gut epithelium in the rat. *J. Physiol. Pharmacol.* 48:719–20.

11. Gilliland, S. E. and M. L. Speck. 1977. Antagonistic action of *Lactobacillus acidophilus* toward intestinal and foodborne pathogens associative cultures. *J. Food Prot.* 40:820–23.

12. Fernandes, C. F., K. M. Shahani, and M. A. Amer. 1987. Therapeutic role of dietary lactobacilli and lactobacillic fermented dairy products. *FEMS Microbiol. Rev.* 46:343–56.

13. Rasic, J. L. and J. A. Kurmann. *Birkhauser Verlag.* Basel, 1983.

14. Polonskaya, M. S. 1952. Antibiotic from acidophilus. *Mikrobiologiya* 21:303–10.

15. Barone, F. E. and M. R. Tansey. 1977. Isolation, purification, identification, synthesis, and kinetics of activity of *allium sativum*, and a hypothesis for its mode of action, *Mycologia* 69:793–825.

16. Reddy, G. V., K. M. Shahani, B. A. Friend, and R. C. Chandan. 1983. Natural antibiotic activity of *Lactobacillus acidophilus* and *bulgaricus* III. Production and partial purification of bulgarican from *Lactobacillus bulgaricus*. *Cult. Dairy Prod. J.* 18:15–19.

17. Ahmed, A. A., R. D. McCarthy, and G. A. Porter. 1979. Effect of milk constituents on hepatic cholesterogenesis. *Atherosclerosis* 32:347–57.

18. *Alternative Medicine—The Definitive Guide.* Everything you must know about effective therapies and affordable self-help cures for you and your family. Compiled by The Burton Goldberg Group.

19. Shahani, K. M., J. R. Vakil, and R. C. Chandan. 1972. Antibiotic acidophilin and process of preparing the same, US Patent 3,689,640.

20. Zacconi, C., V. Bottazzi, A. Rebecchi, E. Bosi, P. G. Sarra, and L. Tagliaferri. 1992. Serum cholesterol levels in axenic mice colonized with *Enterococcus faecium* and *Lactobacillus acidophilus*. *Microbiologica* 15:413–17.

21. Alm, L. 1983. The effect of *Lactobacillus acidophilus* administration upon survival of *Salmonella* in randomly selected human carriers. *Prog. Food Nutr. Sci.* 7:13–17.

22. Butler, C. and J. W. Beakley. 1960. Bacterial flora in vaginitis. *Am. J. Obstet. Gynecol.* 7:432.

23. Hurley, R., V. C. Stanley, B. G. S. Leask, and J. Delouvois. 1974. Bacteriology of the vagina in 75 normal young adults. *Surg. Gynecol. Obstet.* 87:410.

24. Guillot, N. 1958. Elaboration par *Lactobacillus acidophilus* d'un produit actif contre *Candida albicans*. *Ann. Inst. Pasteur* 95:194–207.

25. Collins, E. B. and P. Hardt. 1980. Inhibition of *Candida albicans* by *Lactobacillus acidophilus*. *J. Dairy Sci.* 63:830–32.

26. Wood, J. R., R. L. Sweet, A. Catena, W. K. Hadley, and M. Robbie. 1985. In vitro adherence of *Lactobacillus* species to vaginal epithelial cells. *Am. J. Obstet. Gynecol.* 153:740–43.

27. Svanborg Eden, C., L. A. Hanson, U. Jodal, U. Lindberg, and S. Akerlund. 1976. Variable adherence to normal human urinary-tract epithelial cells of *Escherichia coli* strains associated with various forms of urinary-tract infections. *Lancet* ii: 490–92.

28. Chan, R. C. Y. and A. W. Bruce. 1983. Influence of growth media on the morphology and in vitro adherence characteristics of Gram-negative urinary pathogens. *J. Urol.* 129:411–17.

29. Reid, G., H. J. L. Brooks, and D. F. Bacon. 1983. *In vitro* attachment of *Escherichia coli* to human uroepithelial cells: variation in receptivity during the menstrual cycle and pregnancy. *J. Infect. Dis.* 148:412–21.

30. Shand, G. H., H. Anwar, H. Kadurugath, M. R. W. Brown, S. H. Silverman, and J. Melling. 1985. *In vivo* evidence that bacteria in urinary tract infection grow under iron restricted conditions. *Infect. Immun.* 48:35–39.

31. Chan, R. C. Y., A. W. Bruce, and G. Reid. 1984. Adherence of cervical, vaginal and distal urethral normal microbial flora to human uroepithelial cells and the inhibition of adherence of Gram-negative uropathogens by competitive exclusion. *J. Urol.* 131:596–601.

32. Hurt, H. D. 1972. Heart disease—Is diet a factor? *J. Milk Food Technol.* 35:340–48.

33. Brown, M. S. and J. L. Goldstein. 1984. How LDL receptors influence cholesterol and atherosclerosis. *Sci. Am.* 251:58–66.

34. Miller, N. E., D. S. Theille, O. H. Forde, and O. D. Mjies. 1977. High density lipoprotein and coronary heart disease: A prospective case-control study. *Lancet* i: 965–68.

35. Gordon, T., W. P. Castelli, M. C. Hjortland, W. B. Kannel, and T. R. Dawber. 1977. High density lipoproteins as a protective factor against coronary heart disease—The Framingham Study. *Am. J. Med.* 62:707–14.

36. Jones, G. Hypercholestermic and hypoglyceridemic effect of acidophilus yogurt. MS thesis, University of Nebraska–Lincoln.

37. Ahmed, A. A., R. D. McCarthy, and G. A. Porter. 1979. Effect of milk constituents on hepatic cholesterogenesis. *Atherosclerosis* 32:347–57.

38. Grunewald, K. K. 1985. Influence of bacterial starter cultures on nutritional value of foods: Effects of *L. acidophilus* fermented milk on growth and serum cholesterol in laboratory animals. *Cult. Dairy Prod. J.* 20(2):26–27.

39. Tortuero, F., A. Brenes, and J. Rioperez. 1975. The influence of intestinal flora on serum cholesterol. *Am. J. Clin. Nutr.* 36:1106–11.

40. Harrison, V. C. and G. Peat. 1975. Serum cholesterol and bowel flora in the newborn. *Am. J. Clin. Nutr.* 28:1351–55.

41. Shahani, K. M. and K. C. Chandan. 1979. Nutritional and healthful aspects of cultured and culture-containing dairy foods. *J. of Dairy Sci.* 62:1685–94.

42. Zychowicz, C., A. Surazynska, and T. Cieplinska. 1974. Effect of *Lactobacillus acidophilus* cultures (acidophilus milk) on the carrier state of *Shigella* and *Salmonella* organisms in children. *Ped. Pol.* 49:997–1003.

43. Alm, L. 1983. The effect of *Lactobacillus acidophilus* administration upon survival of *Salmonella* in randomly selected human carriers. *Prog. Food Nutr. Sci.* 7:13–17.

44. Kenworthy, R. and I. Mitchell. 1976. *Escherichia coli* infection of gnotobiotic pigs: Significance of enterotoxin and endotoxin in the clinical state. *J. Comp. Patho.* 86:27–84.

45. Vanderhoof, J. A., D. B. Whitney, D. L. Antonson, T. L. Hanner, J. V. Lupo, and R. J. Young. 1999. Lactobacillus GG in the prevention of antibiotic-associated diarrhea in children. *J. Pediatr.* 135:564–68.

46. Nelson, R. R. 1999. Intrinsically vancomycin-resistant Gram-positive organisms: Clinical relevance and implications for infection control. *J. Hosp. Infect.* 42:275–82.

47. Tomic-Karovic, K. and J. J. Fanjek. 1962. Acidophilus milk in therapy of infantile diarrhea caused by pathogenic *Escherichia coli. Ann. Pediatr.* 199:625–34.

48. Malakar, P. K., D. E. Martens, M. H, Zwietering, C. Beal, and K. van't Riet. 1999. Modelling the interactions between *Lactobacillus curvatus* and *Enterobacter cloacae.* II. Mixed cultures and shelf life predictions. *Int. J. Food Microbiol.* 51:67–79.

49. Fernandes, C. F., R. C. Chandan, and K. M. Shahani. 1992. Fermented dairy products and health, in *Lactic Acid Bacteria*, vol. 1, (B. J. B. Wood, ed.). Elsevier Publishing House, London, pp. 297–339.

50. Ratcliffe, B., C. B. Cole, R. Fuller, and M. J. Newport. 1986. The effect of yogurt and milk fermented with a porcine intestinal strain of *Lactobacillus rueteri* on the performance and gastrointestinal flora of pigs weaned at two days of age. *Food Microbiology* 3:203–11.

51. Fernandes, C. F., R. C. Chandan, and K. M. Shahani. 1992. Fermented dairy products and health, in *Lactic Acid Bacteria*, vol. 1, (B. J. B. Wood, ed.). Elsevier Publishing House, London, pp. 297–339.

52. Fernandes, C. F. and K. M. Shahani. 1989. Modulation of antibiosis by lactobacilli and yogurt and its healthful and beneficial significance. *Proceedings of National Yogurt Association.* New York, NY, pp. 145–59.

53. Reddy, G. V., K. M. Shahani, and M. R. Banerjee. 1973. Effect of yogurt on Ehrlich ascites tumor-cell profileration. *J. Nat'l Cancer Inst.* 50:815–17.

54. Clemmesen, J. 1989. Antitumor effect of lactobacilli substances: *L. bulgaricus* effect. *Mol. Biother.* 1(5):279–82.

55. Bogdanov, I. G., P. G. Dalev, A. I. Gurevich, M. N. Kolosov, V. P. Mal'Kova, L. A. Plemyannikova, and I. B. Sorokina. 1975. Antitumor glycopeptides from *Lactobacillus bulgaricus* cell wall. *FEBS Lett.* 57:259.

56. Reddy, G. V., K. M. Shahani, and M. R. Banerjee. 1973. Effect of yogurt on Ehrlich ascites tumor-cell profileration. *J. Nat'l Cancer Inst.* 50:815–17.

57. Mizutani, T. and T. Mitsuoka. 1988. Effect of dietary phenobarbital on spontaneous hepatic tumorigenesis in germfree C3H/He male mice. *Cancer Lett.* 39:233–37.

58. Shahani, K. M., C. F. Fernandes, and M. A. Amer. 1987. Effect of yogurt on intestinal flora and immune responses. *Proc. Symp. On Yogurt,* Union of Belguim Dairy Industry, pp. 57–67.

59. Sekine, K., J. Ohta, M. Onishi, T. Tatsuki, Y. Shimokawa, T. Toida, T. Kawashima, and Y. Hashimoto. 1995. Analysis of antitumor

properties of effector cells stimulated with a cell wall preparation (WPG) of *Bifidobacterium infantis*. *Biol. Pharm. Bull.* 18:148–53.

60. Ayebo, A. D., I. A. Angelo, and K. M. Shahani. 1981. Effect of ingesting *Lactobacillus acidophilus* milk upon fecal flora and enzyme activity in humans. *Milchwissenschaft* 35:730–33.

61. Dodds, K. L. and D. L. Collins-Thompson. 1984. Incidence of nitrite-depleting lactic acid bacteria in cured meats and in starter cultures. *J. Food Prot.* 47:7–10.

62. Dodds, K. L. and D. L. Collins-Thompson. 1985. Characteristics of nitrite reductase activity in *Lactobacillus lactis* TS4. *Can. J. Microbiol.* 31:558–62.

63. Goldin, B. R., L. Swenson, J. Dwyer, M. Sexton, and S. L. Gorbach. 1980. Effect of diet and *Lactobacillus acidophilus* supplements on human fecal bacterial enzymes. *J. Nat'l Cancer Inst.* 64:255–61.

64. Goldin, B. R. and S. L. Gorbach. 1984. The effect of milk and lactobacillus feeding on human intestinal bacterial enzyme activity. *Am. J. Clin. Nutr.* 39:756–61.

65. Sinha, D. K. 1979. Development of a Nonfermented Acidophilus Milk and Testing its Properties. MS thesis, University of Nebraska–Lincoln.

66. Williams, J. R., P. M. Grantham, H. H. Marsh III, J. H. Weisburger, and E. K. Weisburger. 1970. Participation of liver fraction and of intestinal bacteria in the metabolism of N-hydrexy N-2 fluorenylacetamide in the rat. *Biochem. Pharmacol.* 19:173–88.

67. Roed, T. O. and T. Medtvedt. 1977. Origin of intestinal β-glucuronidase in germ-free, monocontaminated and conventional rats. *Acta. Path. Microbiol. Scand. Sect. B. Microbiol.* 85:271–76.

68. Kent, T. H., L. J. Fischer, and R. Marr. 1972. Glucuronidase activity in intestinal contents of rats and man and relationship to bacterial flora. *Proc. Soc. Exp. Biol. Med.* 140:590–94.

69. Hawksworth, G., B. S. Drasar, and M. J. Hill. 1971. Intestinal bacteria and the hydrolysis of glycosidic bounds. *J. Med. Microbiol.* 4:451–59.

70. Gadeile, D., P. Raibaud, and E. Sacquet. 1985. β-glucuronidase activities of intestinal bacteria determined both in vitro and in vivo gnotobiotic rats. *Appl. Environ. Microbiol.* 49:682–85.

71. Kato, I., S. Kobayashi, T. Yokokura, and M. Mutai. 1981. Anti-tumor activity of *Lactobacillus casei* in mice. *Gann.* 72:517–23.

72. Kato, I., T. Yokokura, and M. Mutai. 1983. Macrophage activation by *Lactobacillus casei* in mice. *Microbiol. Immunol.* 27:611–18.

73. Bogdanov, I. G., P. G. Dalev, A. I. Gurevich, M. N. Kolosov, V. P. Mal'Kova, L. A. Plemyannikova, and I. B. Sorokina. 1975. Antitumor glycopeptides from *Lactobacillus bulgaricus* cell wall. *FEBS Lett.* 57:259.

74. Friend, B. A., R. E. Farmer, and K. M. Shahani. 1982. Effect of feeding and intraperitoneal implantation of yogurt culture cells on Ehrlich ascites tumor cells. *Milchwissenschaft* 37:708–10.

75. Kohwi, Y., K. Imai, Z. Tamura, and Y. Hasimoto. 1978. Anti-tumor effect of *Bifidobacterium infantis* in mice. *Gann.* 69:613–18.

76. Kohwi, Y., Y. Hashimoto, and Z. Tamura. 1982. Anti-tumor and immunological adjuvant effect of *Bifidobacterium infantis* in mice. *Bifidobact. Microfl.* 1:61.

77. Kohwi, Y., K. Imai, Z. Tamura, and Y. Hasimoto. 1978. Anti-tumor effect of *Bifidobacterium infantis* in mice. *Gann.* 69:613–18.

78. Kohwi, Y., Y. Hashimoto, and Z. Tamura. 1982. Anti-tumor and immunological adjuvant effect of *Bifidobacterium infantis* in mice. *Bifidobact. Microfl.* 1:61.

79. Hosono, A. and T. Kashina. 1986. Antimutagenic properties of lactic acid cultured milk on chemical and fecal mutagens. *J. Dairy Sci.* 69:2237–42.

80. Mayer, J. B. 1969. Interrelationships between diet, intestinal flora and viruses. *Phys. Med. Rehabilitation* 10(1):16–23.

81. Tihole, F. 1988. Possible treatment of AIDS patients with live lactobacteria. *Medical Hypothesis* 26:85–88.

82. Cummings, J. H. and G. T. Macfarlane. 1997. Role of intestinal bacteria in nutrient metabolism. *JPEN J. Parenter. Enteral. Nutr.* 21:357–65.

83. Gallop, P. M., J. B. Lian, and P. V. Hauschka. 1980. Carboxylated calcium-binding proteins and vitamin K, *NE JM* 302:1460–66.

84. Kaup, S. M., K. M. Shahani, and M. A. Amer. 1987. Bioavailability of calcium in yogurt. *Milchwissenschaft* 42:518.

85. Perdigon, G., E. Vintini, S. Alvarez, M. Medina, and M. Medici. 1999. Study of the possible mechanisms involved in the mucosal immune system activation by lactic acid bacteria. *J. Dairy Sci.* 82:1108–14.

86. Shahani, K. M., C. F. Fernandes, and M. A. Amer. 1988. Immunologic and therapeutic modulation of gastrointestinal microecology by lactobacilli. *Microbiol. and Therapy* 18:103–4.

87. Van de Water, J., C. I. Keen, and M. E. Gershwin. 1999. The influence of chronic yogurt consumption on immunity. *J. Nutr.* 129:1492S–95S.

88. Perdigon, G., M. E. Nader de Macias, S. Alverez, G. Oliver, and A. A. Pesce de Ruiz Holgado. 1987. Enhancement of immune responses in mice fed with *Streptococcus thermophilus* and *Lactobacillus acidophilus. J. of Dairy Sci.* 70:919–26.

89. Lipkin, M. and H. Newmark. 1985. Effect of added dietary calcium on colonic epithelial cell proliferation in subjects with high risk for familiar colonic cancer. *N. England J. Med.* 313:1381–84.

90. Paryavi-Gholami, F., G. E. Minah, and B. F. Turng. 1999. Oral malodor in children and volatile sulfur compound-producing bacteria in saliva: Preliminary microbiological investigation. *Pediatr. Dent.* 21:320–24.

91. Johansson, M. L., S. Nobaek, A. Berggren, M. A. Nyman, I. Bjorck, S. Ahrne, B. Jeppsson, and G. Molin. 1998. Survival of *Lactobacillus*

*plantarum* DSM 9843 (299v), and effect on the short-chain fatty acid content of faeces after ingestion of a rose-hip drink with fermented oats. *Int. J. Food Microbiol.* 42:29–38.

92. Friend, B. A., J. M. Fiedler, and K. M. Shahani. 1983. Influence of culture selection on the flavor, antimicrobial activity, Beta-galactosidase and B-vitamin of yogurt. *Milchwissenschaft* 38:133–36.

93. Rao, D. R. and K. M. Shahani. 1987. Vitamin content of cultured dairy products. *Cult. Dairy Prod.* 22(1):6–10.

94. Gallop, P. M., J. B. Lian, and P. V. Hauschka. 1980. Carboxylated calcium-binding proteins and vitamin K, *NE JM* 302:1460–66.

95. Von Wright, A. and S. Salminen. 1999. Probiotics: Established effects and open questions. *Eur. J. Gastroenterol. Hepatol.* 11:1195–98.

96. Sanders, M. E. and J. Huis in't Veld. 1999. Bringing a probiotic-containing functional food to the market: microbiological, product, regulatory and labeling issues. *Antonie Van Leeuwenhoek,* 76:293–315.

97. Fernandez, C. F., K. M. Shahani, and M. A. Amer. 1988. Control of diarrhea by lactobacilli. *J. of App. Nutr.* 40(1):32–42.

98. Speck, M. L. 1976. Interactions among lactobacilli and man. *J. Dairy Sci.* 59:338–43.

99. Salminen, S., E. Isolauri, and T. Onnela. 1995. Gut flora in normal and disordered states. *Chemotherapy* 41:5–15.

100. Cohendy, M. 1906. Essais d'acclimation microbiene dans la cavity intestinale. *C. R. Soc. Bull.* Paris, 60:364.

101. Black, F. T., K. Einarsson, A. Lidbeck, K. Orrhage, and C. Nord. 1991. Effects of lactic acid producing bacteria on the human intestinal micoflora during ampicillin treatment. *Scand. J. Infect. Dis.* 23:247–54.

102. Niv, M., W. Levy, and N. M. Greenstein. 1963. Yogurt in the treatment of infantile diarrhea. *Clin. Ped.* 2:407.

103. Butel, M. J., N. Roland, A. Hibert, F. Popot, A. Favre, A. C. Tessedre, M. Bensaada, A. Raimbault, and O. Szylit. 1998. Clostridial pathogenity in experimental necrotising enterocolitis in gnotobiotic quails and protective role of bifidobacteria. *J. Med. Microbiol.* 47:391–99.

104. Urao, M., T. Fujimoto, G. J. Lane, G. Seo, and T. Miyano. 1999. Does probiotics administration decrease serum endotoxin levels in infants? *J. Pediatr. Sug.* 34:273–76.

105. Ferrer, F. P., and L .J. Boyd. 1955. Effect of yogurt with prune whip on constipation. *Am. J. Dog. Dis.* 22:272.

106. Teuri, U. and R. Korpela. 1998. Galacto-oligosaccharides relieve constipation in elderly people. *Ann. Nutr. Metab.* 42:273–76.

107. Schmidt, W. U., J. Sattler, R. Hesterberg, H. D. Roher, T. Zoedler, H. Sitter, and W. Lorenz. 1990. Human intestinal diamine oxidase (DAO)

activity in Crohn's disease: A new marker for disease assessment? *Agents Actions* 30:267–70.

108. Skelton, W. P., III and N. K. Skelton. 1989. Thiamine deficiency neuropathy. It's still common today. *Postgrad. Med.* 85:301–6.

109. Rowland, I. R. and R. Tanaka. 1993. The effects of transgalactosylated oligosaccharides on gut flora metabolism in rats associated with a human faecal microflora. *J. Appl. Bacteriol.* 74:667–74.

110. Classen, J., C. Belka, F. Paulsen, W. Budach, W. Hoffmann, and M. Bamberg. 1998. Radiation-induced gastrointestinal toxicity. Pathophysiology approaches to treatment and prophylaxis. *Strahlenther Onkol.* 174:82–84.

111. *International Dermatology News*, 1988, vol 21, no. 3.

112. Meinhof, W. and F. Schropl. 1974. Incidence of pathogenic dermatophytes in patients of a super-regional diagnostic hospital. A contribution to the epidemiology of skin mycoses. *Hautarzt.* 25:139–42.

113. Toivanen, P., D. S. Hansen, F. Mestre, L. Lehtonen, J. Vaahtovuo, M. Vehma, T. Mottonen, R. Saario, R. Luukkainen, and M. Nissila. 1999. Somatic serogroups, capsular types, and species of fecal Klebsiella in patients with ankylosing spondylitis. *J. Clin. Microbiol.* 37:1808–12.

114. Coconnier, M. H., V. Lievin, M. F. Bernet-Camard, S. Hudault, and A. L. Servin. 1997. Antibacterial effect of the adhering human *Lactobacillus acidophilus* strain LB. *Antimicrob. Agents Chemother.* 41:1046–52.

115. Kjeldsen-Kragh, J. 1999. Rhematoid arthritis treated with vegetarian diets. *Am. J. Clin. Nutr.* 70:594S–600S.

116. Underdahl, N. R. 1983. The effect of feeding *Streptococcus faecium* upon *Escherichia coli* induced diarrhea in gnotobiotic pigs. *Prog. Food Nutr. Sci.* 7:5–12.

117. Lewenstein, A., G. Frigerio, and M. Moroni. 1979. Biological properties of *Streptococcus faecium*, a new approach for the treatment of diarrheal diseases. *Curr. Ther. Res.* 26:967–81.

118. Chandan, R. C. 1999. Enhancing market value of milk by adding cultures. *J. Dairy Sci.* 82:2245–56.

119. Shahani, K. M. From a lecture given at Optimal Health Systems, Mesa, Arizona, 1985.

120. Saavedra, J. M. 1999. Probiotics plus antibiotics: regulating our bacterial environment. *J. Pediatr.* 135:535–37.

121. Toivanen, P., D. S. Hansen, F. Mestre, L. Lehtonen, J. Vaahtovuo, M. Vehma, T. Mottonen, R. Saario, R. Luukkainen, and M. Nissila. 1999. Somatic serogroups, capsular types, and species of fecal Klebsiella in patients with ankylosing spondylitis. *J. Clin. Microbiol.* 37:1808–12.

# The Candida Epidemic

1. Belem, M. A. and B. H. Lee. 1998. Production of bioingredients from *Kluyeromyces marxianus* grown on whey: An alternative. *Crit. Rev. Food Sci. Nutr.* 38:565–98.

2. Bryant, K., C. Maxfield, and G. Rabalais. 1999. Renal candidiasis in neonates with candiduria. *Pediatr. Infect. Dis. J.* 18:959–63.

3. Brown, A. J. and N. A. Gow. 1999. Regulatory networks controlling *Candida albicans* morphogenesis. *Trends Microbiol.* 7:333–38.

4. Girishkumar, H., A. M. Yousuf, J. Chivate, and E. Geisler. 1999. Experience with invasive candida infections. *Postgrad. Med. J.* 75:151–53.

5. Opaneye, A. A. 1999. Genital thrush in women: The attitudes and practice patterns of general practitioners in Teesside and north Yorkshire. *J.R. Soc. Health* 119:163–65.

6. Scheutz, F., M. I., Matee, E. Simon, J. H. Mwinula, E. F. Lyamuya, A. E. Msengi, and L. P. Samaranayake. 1997. Association between carriage of oral yeasts, malnutrition and HIV-1 infection among Tanzanian children aged 18 months to 5 years. *Community Dent. Oral Epidemiol.* 25:193–98.

7. Knoke, M., K. Schulz, and H. Bernhardt. 1997. Dynamics of candida isolations from humans from 1992–1995 in Greifswald, Germany. *Mycoses* 40:105–10.

8. Abu-Elteen, K. H. 1999. Incidence and distribution of candida species isolated from human skin in Jordan. *Mycoses* 42:311–17.

9. Niimi, M., R. D. Cannon, and B. C. Monk. 1999. *Candida albicans* pathogenicity: A proteomic perspective. *Electrophoresis* 20:2299–2308.

10. Girishkumar, H., A. M. Yousuf, J. Chivate, and E. Geisler. 1999. Experience with invasive candida infections. *Postgrad. Med. J.* 75:151–53.

11. Rangavajhyala, N., K. M. Shahani, G. Sridevi, and S. Srikumaran. 1997. Non-Lipolysaccharide component(s) of *Lactobacillus acidophilus* stimulate(s) the production of interleukin-1-alpha by murine macrophages. *Nutrition and Cancer* 27:130–34.

12. Hilton, E., H. D. Isenberg, P. Alperstein, K. France, and M. T. Borenstein. 1992. Ingestion of yogurt-containing *Lactobacillus acidophilus* as prophylaxis for candidal vaginitis. *An. of Int. Med.* 116:353–57.

13. Murray, F. 1990. Better nutrition for today's living. *Lancet* 52:14.

14. Fredricsson, B., K. Englund, C. E. Nord, and L. Weintraub. 1992. Could bacterial vaginosis be due to the competitive suppression of lactobacilli by aerobic microorganisms? *Gynecol. Obstet. Invest.* 33:119–23.

15. Robertson, J., W. G. Brydon, K. Tadesse, P. Wenham, A. Walls, and M. A. Eastwood. 1979. The effect of raw carrot on serum lipids and colon function. *Am. J. Clin. Nutr.* 32:1889–92.

16. Enderlein, Gunther. 1981. Bakterien—cycologenie, Semmelweis Institute.

17. Hilton, E., H. D. Isenberg, P. Alperstein, K. France, and M. T. Borenstein. 1992. Ingestion of yogurt containing *Lactobacillus acidophilus* as prophylaxix for candidal vaginitis. *Ann. Intern. Med.* 116:353–57.

## Lactose Intolerance

1. Pochart, P., P. Marteau, Y. Bouhnik, I. Goderel, P. Bourlioux, and J. C. Rambaud. 1992. Survival of bifidobacteria ingested via fermented milk during their passage through the human small intestine: An in vivo study using intestinal perfusion. *Am. J. Clin. Nutr.* 55:78–80.

## Are All Probiotics Alike?

1. Bastos, M. C., P. J. Mondino, M. L. Azevedo, K. R. Santos, and M. Giambaigi-deMarval. 1999. Molecular characterization and transfer among staphylococcus strains of a plasmid conferring high level resistance to mupirocin. *Eur. J. Clin. Microbiol. Infect. Dis.* 18:393–98.

2. Gilliland, S. E. and M. L. Speck. 1977. Enumeration and identity of lactobacilli in dietary products. *J. Food Prot.* 40:760–62.

3. Brennan, M., B. Wanismail, and B. Ray. 1983. Prevalence of viable *Lactobacillus acidophilus* in dried commercial products. *J. Food Prot.* 46:887–92.

4. Lee, Y.-K. and S. Salminen. 1996. The coming of age of probiotics. *Trends in Food Sci. Technol.* 6:241–45.

5. Goldin, B. R., S. L. Gorbach, M. Saxelin, S. Barakat, L. Gualtieri, and S. Salminen. 1992. Survival of lactobacillus species in human gastrointestinal tract. *Dig. Dis. Sci.* 37:121–28.

6. Voragen, A. G. J. 1998. Technological aspects of functional food-related carbohydrates. *Trends in Food Sci. & Tech.* 9:328–35.

7. Kilara, A., K. M. Shahani, and N. K. Das. 1976. Effect of cryoprotective agents on freeze-drying and storage of lactic cultures. *Cult. Dairy Prod. J.* 11:8–12.

## Using Probiotics Throughout the Life Span

1. Petersdorf, R. G. *Principles of Internal Medicine.* McGraw Hill Publications, New York, 1983, pp. 359–60.

2. Bennet, P. 1991. *Vegetarian Times* 167:14.

3. Bullen, C. I., A. T. Willis, and K. Williams. 1973. The significance of bifidobacteria in the intestinal tract of infants. *Soc. Appl. Bacteriol. Symp. Ser.* 2:211–325.

# Glossary of Key Words

Terms defined in this glossary introduce each entry and appear in boldface. Within entries, other terms that are also defined in the glossary are bold and underscored.

**acid-fast** Refers to a **microorganism** that is not readily decolorized by **acids** when stains are applied.

**acetic acid** A saturated fatty acid. It is the characteristic component of vinegar.

**acidophilin** A natural antibioticlike substance elaborated by *L. Acidophilus,* also called a "bacterocin."

**acids** [Latin *acere,* to be sour] In biochemistry, a substance which, due to its makeup, is able to give up a hydrogen to another kind of substance (a base which, due to its makeup, can accept a hydrogen atom).

**acne** An inflammatory disease of the glands in the skin.

**adrenal hormones** Chemical substances, produced by the adrenal glands, that get secreted into the blood and sent to other cells and organs to cause specific effects on them.

**aerobic** A life form that requires oxygen in order to live, or a condition that has and/or needs oxygen available.

**allergic** A hypersensitive reactive condition that occurs upon exposure to a specific substance.

**allicin** The volatile sulfur-containing compound in garlic that is primarily responsible for its pungent smell, but is, in fact, also responsible for most of its pharmacological and beneficial properties (lowering of cholesterol levels and blood pressure).

**amazake** Literally "sweet sake," this product is made from fermented rice. It is a creamy-thick hot drink that has a rich ambrosial flavor and virtually no alcohol content. A specialty in Japanese teahouses and inns.

**ambient** [Latin *ambi,* around + *ire,* to go] Surrounding; on all sides.

**amino acids** The building blocks that make up proteins.

**amylase** An enzyme that helps change starch or complex carbohydrates into smaller units of sugar. It is found in saliva, pancreatic juice, and in certain raw foods.

**anaerobic** A life form that does not require oxygen and survives without it, or a condition that does not have and/or need oxygen available.

**anticarcinogenic** A substance that is shown to contribute to the prevention, destruction, or suppression of a tendency to develop cancer.

**antibodies** Protein molecules produced in the body that have a specific **amino acid** sequence that interacts with a specific **antigen** when it comes into contact with the body , neutralizing it so the antigen can't affect the body.

**antigen** An enzyme, toxin, or other substance, usually of high molecular weight, to which the body reacts by producing antibodies to eliminate it or defend against it.

**antimutagenic** A substance or quality of a substance that can antagonize the **mutagenic** effects of other substances.

**antibiotic** Any of certain chemical substances produced by various **micro-organisms**, or synthetically in a lab, that has the capacity to destroy or inhibit the growth of other bacteria or microorganisms.

**antispasmatic** An agent that relieves **spasm**, usually in smooth muscle such as in arteries, bronchi, intestines, bile ducts, ureters or sphincters, but also may relieve spasm in voluntary muscle.

**antioxidant** One of the many widely used synthetic or natural substances added to a product to prevent or delay its deterioration by oxygen in the air.

**arterial** Referring to the **arteries** of the body.

**arteries** The vessels in the body that are connected to the heart as their central organ. They carry the blood of the heart away from the heart and to the cells of the body and deliver $O_2$ and nutrients to the cells.

**arteriosclerosis** Thickening and loss of elasticity of **artery** walls.

**ascites** [Greek *askos*, bag] Abnormal effusion and accumulation of fluid in the abdominal cavity.

**atherosclerosis** An extremely common form of **arteriosclerosis** in which deposits of yellowish placque, containing cholesterol and fat material, are formed within the layers of large- and medium-sized arteries.

**atherosclerotic** Referring to an artery that has **atherosclerosis**. These deposits are called **atherosclerotic** placques.

**athlete's foot** A chronic fungal infection of the skin of the foot, especially between the toes and on the soles. There may be cracking, scaling, and itching of the skin of the foot.

**atopic eczema** Referring to hypersensitivity or an allergic type of eczema.

**augment** To become bigger or better; to add to something, increasing it.

**aureomycin** Trademark name for preparations of crystalline chlortetracycline hydrochloride (an antibiotic).

**autonomic nervous system** The portion of the nervous system concerned with regulation of the activity of cardiac muscle, smooth muscle, and glands.

**autosomal dominant trait** An autosome is an ordinary paired **chromosome** in animal cells. Humans normally have 46 chromosomes, or 23 pairs (22 autosome pairs and 1 sex pair, either XX or XY, which determines the sex of the organism). The **autosomal dominant trait** is the trait on a chromosome of a pair that exerts a ruling or controlling influence. In genetics, capable of expressing dominance over the other corresponding trait of chromosomes of that pair.

*β*-**galactosidase** an **enzyme** that occurs in the **kidney**, liver, and intestinal mucosa; hydrolyzes the conversion of *β*-D-galactoside to D-galactoside (see **lactase**).

**B$_{12}$** Refers to one of the B vitamins, also called cyanocobalamin. B$_{12}$ is needed for healthy red blood cells.

**B$_6$** Refers to one of the B vitamins, also called **pyridoxine**. It is essential for energy production from **amino acids** and can be considered an "energy-releasing" vitamin.

**bacteria/bacterial** These terms refer to **microorganisms** that are not blue-green algae and/or have a true cell wall surrounding them.

**bacteriocidal** [Latin *caedere*, to kill] Something that is destructive to **bacteria**.

**bacteriostatic** [Greek *stasis*, stoppage] Something that inhibits the growth of **bacteria** but doesn't kill it.

**bacteroides** A genus of nonsporulating, obligate, anaerobic filamentous bacteria occurring as normal flora in the mouth and large bowel; often found in necrotic tissue. Thirty species have been described.

**benzoic acid** An acid, $C_6H_6$ (COOH), in the form of white crystals, scales, or needles made from benzoin (a vegetable or tree resin) and other resins from coal tar that is used as an antifungal agent in pharmaceutical preparations and in combination with salicylic acid as a topical fungal agent.

**bifidobacterium** A **genus** of **anaerobic** lactobacilli.

*Bifidobacterium infantis* (or *B. infantis*) A commonly used form of bifidobacterium.

**bile** A fluid secreted by the liver and poured into the small intestine via the bile ducts. It is concentrated in the gall bladder.

**biliary steroids** Biliary pertains to the **bile**, the bile ducts, or the gall bladder. Bliliary steroids are bile lipids (fats) that have a specific chemical configuration. For details on this configuration, consult a chemistry book.

**bioactivity** Activity caused by a substance that has an effect on, or elicits a response from, living tissue.

**bioavailability** The degree to which a drug or other substance becomes available to the target tissue after administration.

**biosynthesis** The building up of a chemical compound in the physiologic processes of a living organism.

**BUN** (**B**lood **U**rea **N**itrogen) The nitrogen component of <u>urea</u>. The concentration of urea nitrogen in the blood. **BUN** is measured in the determination of <u>kidney</u> function; elevated levels of **BUN** indicate a disorder of kidney function (see <u>urea</u>).

**cancer** [Latin *cancer*, crab] A cellular <u>tumor</u> or abnormal growth, the natural course of which is fatal. **Cancer** cells, unlike benign tumor cells, exhibit the properties of invasion and spread from one location to another.

*Candida albicans* A yeast <u>microorganism</u> found in the normal human organism. It is concentrated on the skin and mucus membranes. Overgrowth of candida is called candidiasis.

**carcinogen** Any <u>cancer</u>-producing substance.

**carcinogenesis** The production of carcinoma (a malignant <u>cancer</u> growth).

**catalyze** [Greek *katalysis*, dissolution].To cause or produce <u>catalysis</u>.

**catalysis** An increase in the velocity of a chemical reaction or process, brought about by the presence of a substance that is not consumed in the net chemical reaction or process.

*C. botulinum* The causative agent of botulism, a type of food poisoning from improperly canned or preserved foods.

**celiac disease** [Greek *koilice*, belly] A disease pertaining to the abdominal organs, specifically, a malabsorption syndrome precipitated by the ingestion of gluten-containing foods; also called **Celiac Sprue**.

**Celiac Sprue** A chronic form of malabsorption syndrome (see **celiac disease**).

**cell membrane** (also known as plasma membrane) The structure enveloping a cell, enclosing the cytoplasm, and forming a selective permeability barrier. It consists of lipids, proteins, and some carbohydrates. The lipids are thought to form a bilayer in which integral proteins are embedded to varying degrees.

**cellular mediated immune system** Refers to a specific, acquired type of immunity in which the role of small lymphocytes of thymic (thymus gland) origin, called T-Lymphocytes, are predominant. Cell-mediated immunity is responsible for resistance to infectious diseases caused by certain bacteria, fungi, and viruses; certain aspects of resistance to cancer; delayed hyper-sensitivity reactions; certain autoimmune diseases; and allograft rejection. It also plays a role in certain allergies.

**cell wall**  A rigid structure that lies just outside of, and is joined to, the plasma membrane of plant cells and most bacteria cells. It protects the cell and maintains its shape.

**centrifugation**  The process of separating the lighter portions of a solution, mixture, or suspension from the heavier portions by spinning the solution fast (centrifugal force).

**centrifuge**  [Latin *fugere*, to flee] A machine used to perform **centrifugation**; or to subject something to **centrifugation**.

**chemotherapeutic drugs**  Chemical agents used to treat disease; first applied to the use of chemicals that affect the causative organisms unfavorably, but do not harm the patient.

**cholesterol**  A substance found in all cells of the body that helps to carry fats. Too much is thought to be bad for the health of the **arteries**.

**chromosome**  A structure in the nucleus that contains a linear-shaped thread of DNA which transmits genetic information. Each organism of a species is normally characterized by the same number of **chromosomes** in its cells. In humans, the normal number is 46, or 23 pairs (22 **autosome** pairs and 1 sex pair either XX or XY, which determines the sex of the organisms), as distinguished from a sex **chromosome**.

**circumvent**  To avoid or defeat, as if by passing around, especially as the result of cleverness.

**clostridium**  [Greek *kloster*, spindle] A type of rod-shaped bacteria that is obligate **anaerobic**, or microaerophilic, Gram-positive, spore-forming. Some 205 species have been identified (e.g., *C. botulinum*, is the agent that causes botulism, a type of food poisoning from improperly canned or preserved food).

**clot**  A semisolid mass, as of blood or lymph.

**coenzyme**  A substance that assists **enzymes** in performing their functions.

**coliform**  [Latin *colum*, a sieve] A collective term referring to intestinal fermentative, Gram-negative bacterial rods, and sometimes restricted to the lactose-forming bacilli (e.g., *Escherichia coli*, Klebsiella, Enterobacter, and Cifrobacter). Any organism of that group is a **coliform** organism.

**coliform count**  Refers to taking an actual quantitative count of the **coliform** organisms present in a culture.

**colonization**  The development of cells in a part to which they have been carried, as in a culture-growing medium.

**colostrum**  The thin, yellow, milky fluid secreted by the mammary gland a few days before or after delivery of a baby. It contains up to 20 percent protein, including immoglobulins, representing the antibodies found in maternal blood. **Colostrum** contains more minerals and less fat and carbohydrates than milk.

**Corynebacterium**  [Greek *koryn*, club + *bakteriun*, little rod] A **genus** of **microorganisms** of the family Corynebacteriaceae, made up of straight to slightly curved rods that are generally aerobic but may be microaerophilic or even anaerobic. To date, 144 species have been described.

**congenital**  [Latin *ccongenitus*, born together] Existing at and usually before birth; referring to conditions that are present at birth, regardless of their causation.

**constituent**  Any of the parts, or one of the parts, that make up a whole.

**coronary heart disease**  A pathology involving the arteries that supply the heart muscle.

**creatine**  [Greek *kreas*, flesh] A crystallizable nitrogenous compound synthesized in the body that is an important storage form of high-energy phosphate.

**creatinine**  An anhydride of **creatine**; the end-product of creatine metabolism; found in muscle and blood and excreted in the urine.

**cryoprotective**  [Greek *kryos*, cold] Capable of protecting against injury due to freezing.

**crystal**  [Greek *krystallos*, ice] A naturally produced, angular solid of definite form in which the ultimate units from which it is built are systematically arranged—evenly arranged on a regular-spaced lattice.

**crystallization**  The formation of **crystals**.

**crystallized**  Something that has formed **crystals**.

**culture**  The propagation of **microorganisms** or living tissue cells in a special medium conducive to their growth. Also, a growth of microorganisms or other living cells.

**cultured**  **Microorganisms** or living cells that have been grown in a special medium.

**culture medium**  Any substance or preparation used for the cultivation of **microorganisms** of living cells.

**D(–) (dextrorotatory)**  [Latin *dexte*, right + *rotare*, to turn] A substance that turns the plane of polarization, or rays of light that pass through it, to the right.

**decolorized**  Something from which all color has been subtracted; bleached.

**diabetic neuropathy** [Greek *diabetes*, a syphon] Diabetes is a general term referring to disorders characterized by excessive urine excretion. **Diabetic neuropathy** is a chronic, symmetrical, sensory functional disturbance and/or pathological change in the nervous system. It first affects the nerves of the lower limbs and often the **autonomic nervous system**.

**dissociate** [Latin *dis*, negative + *sociatio*, union] The act of separating or, by heat, splitting a molecule into two or more simpler molecules.

**DNA** The carrier of genetic information for all organisms except the RNA viruses.

**dormant** [Latin *dormire*, to sleep] Sleeping, or in an inactive state.

**dysbiosis** Abnormal living conditions in the biological system, including the association of dissimilar, noncompatible organisms living in a nonmutually beneficial way; nonconducive to life and destructive to it.

**dysentery** [Greek *dys*, abnormal + *enteron*, intestine] A term given to a number of disorders marked by inflammation of the intestines, especially of the colon, and attended by pain in the abdomen, painful straining at stool or in urination, and frequent stools containing blood and mucus. The causative agent may be chemical irritants, bacteria, protozoa, or parasitic worms.

**eczema** [Greek *ekzein*, to boil out] A superficial inflammation, involving primarily the skin, characterized by redness, itching, papules and vesicles, weeping, oozing, crusting, and later scaling and pigmentation.

**Ehrlich ascites** A type of cancer cell much used in research.

**Ehrlich carcinoma or sarcoma** Types of **cancer**.

**emulsify** To convert or be converted into an emulsion.

**emulsion** A preparation of one liquid distributed in small globules throughout the body of a second liquid.

**enomycin (Kaopectate)** An over-the-counter medication used to stop diarrhea conditions.

**Enterobacterioacae** A family of Gram-negative rod-shaped organisms, occurring as plant or animal parasites, or living upon dead or decaying organic matter. It includes five tribes.

*Enterococci faecium* A *Ptococcus* of the human intestine. It used to be called *Streptococcus faeciuim*. It is a normal inhabitant of the intestinal tract and a cause of subacute bacterial endocarditis.

**enzymatic** Related to, caused by, or of the nature of an **enzyme**.

**enzyme** Proteins that regulate all the body's chemical reactions. In fact, without **enzymes**, no activity at all would take place. There are three categories:

(1) Food **enzymes**, contained in the raw foods we eat; (2) Digestive **enzymes**, made and secreted by the digestive organs in the body; and (3) metabolic **enzymes**, which are all the other enzymes that regulate the body's chemical reactions.

**eosin stain**  [Greek *eos*, dawn] A rose-colored stain or dye.

**epithelial cells**  The cells that make up the **epithelium**.

**epithelium**  [Greek *epi*, on + *thele*, nipple] The covering of internal and external surfaces of the body, including the lining of vessels and other small cavities. It consists of cells joined by small amounts of cementing substances.

*Escherichia*  A **genus** of **microorganisms** made up of Gram-negative, motile or nonmotile short rods, widely distributed in nature and occasionally pathogenic for man.

**essential amino acids**  **Amino acids** are the building blocks of protein. The **essential amino acids** must be taken in daily from the diet because the body does not make them.

**estrogen**  A generic term for the female sex hormones. In humans, estrogen is formed in the ovary, adrenal cortex, testis, and feto-placental unit, and it has various functions in both sexes. It is responsible for development of female secondary sex characteristics.

**etiological**  [Greek *aitia*, cause + *logy*, the study of] Pertaining to the causes of disease.

**facultative**  Not obligatory; pertaining to, or characterized by, the ability to adjust to particular circumstances or to assume a particular role.

**fatty acids**  The building blocks that make up fats.

**fecal**  Pertaining to, or of the nature of, **feces**.

**feces**  [Latin *faex*, refuse] The excrement discharge from the intestines, consisting of bacteria, old intestine cells, secretions—chiefly of the liver— and a small amount of food residue.

**fermentation**  The **anaerobic enzymatic** conversion of organic compounds, especially carbohydrates, to simpler compounds. This results in energy in the form of ATP. It differs from respiration in that organic substances are used rather than molecular oxygen as electron acceptors.

**flora**  The bacteria normally residing within a certain area of the body (e.g., intestinal flora).

**FMP** (**F**ermented **M**ilk **P**roducts)  A derivative of riboflavin (vitamin $B_2$) that acts as a **coenzyme**.

**food sensitivity**  A state or quality of being abnormally sensitive or irritated by a certain food.

**fortuitous** A lucky or fortunate chance happening or accident.

**free radical** A group of atoms that are extremely reactive and carry an unpaired electron.

**gall bladder** The pear-shaped reservoir for the bile on the back, lower surface of the liver. From the gall bladder neck, the cystic duct projects to join the common bile duct.

**gastrointestinal system** The entire digestive system, including all its functional and structural parts from the mouth to the anus.

**genetic** Pertaining to reproduction, or to birth or origin; inherited; referring to a blueprint pattern in a cell.

**genus** (plural, **genera**) A category superior to a species or subspecies and subordinate to a tribe or subtribe.

**globulin** A class of proteins characterized by being insoluble in water, but soluble in saline solutions *or* water-soluble proteins, whose other physical properties resemble the **globulins**.

**glutathione** [Greek *theion*, sulfur] Composed of glutamic acid, cysteine, and aminoacetic acid, and isolated from animal and plant tissues. It is a **coenzyme** and acts as a respiratory carrier of oxygen in cellular reactions, making it an antioxidant.

**gluten** A substance from wheat to which many people have an allergic reaction.

**gnotobiotic** [Greek *gnotos*, known + *biota*, the fauna and flora of a region] Pertaining to a gnotobiote or to **gnotobiotics**.

**gnotobiotics** The science of rearing laboratory animals. Gnotobiotics refers to the microfauna and microflora of an area or region that are specifically known in their entirety.

**Gram stain (Gram-negative, Gram-positive)** Hans Christian Joachim Gram, a Danish physician (1853–1938), devised a staining procedure in which **microorganisms** are stained with crystal violet, treated with a 1:15 dilution of Lugol's iodine, **decolorized** with ethanol or ethanol acetone, and counterstained with contrasting die, usually red safranin. Those **microorganisms** that retain the crystal violet stain are said to be **Gram-positive**, and those that lose the crystal violet stain by decolorization, but stain with the counterstain, are said to be **Gram-negative**. There is no fundamental difference between Gram-positive and Gram-negative organisms; it is merely one way to classify bacteria.

**gut** The intestine or bowel, or digestive tube.

**halitosis** A condition of bad breath.

**HDL** (High-Density Lipoprotein) A blood plasma lipoprotein containing high levels of protein, little triglycerides, moderate levels of phospholipids, and relatively little cholesterol.

**heart attack** An attack/episode of heart dysfunction. It can be mild to severe and life-threatening. The causes can be numerous.

**homeostasis** [Greek *homoios*, like, always the same, unchanging + *stasis*, standing] The maintenance of relatively stable internal physiological conditions (as body temperature or the pH of the blood) in an organism under fluctuating environmental conditions. It is achieved by a system of control mechanisms within an organism.

**hormonal system** A system made up of nine different glands that regulate body activity by their special secretions, the **hormones**, into the bloodstream.

**hormones** [Greek *hormaein*, to set in motion, spur on] A chemical substance produced in the body by an organ or cells of an organ (commonly by an endocrine gland). **Hormones** have a specific regulatory effect on the activity of certain cells and organs.

**host-specific** Characteristic of a particular species or host; having a characteristic effect on, or interaction with, cells or tissues of members of a specific species. May refer to an **antigen**, drug, or infective agent.

**human-specific** When the characteristic effects are on humans only.

**humoral immunity** This is an acquired immunity in which the role of circulating **antibodies** (**immunoglobulins**) is predominant; these antibodies are products of B-lymphocytes and plasma cells.

**hydrogen peroxide** ($H_2O_2$) A strong disinfectant, cleansing, and bleaching liquid used in a diluted solution in water, mainly as a wash or a spray.

**hydrolyze** To subject to **hydrolysis**.

**hydrolysis** The splitting of a compound into fragments by the addition of water, the hydroxyl group (OH) being incorporated into one fragment and the hydrogen (H) atom into the other.

**hypercholesteremia** [Greek *hyper*, above + cholesterol + *haima*, blood] Excess of **cholesterol** in the blood.

**hypertension** Persistently high arterial blood pressure.

**hypocalcemia** Reduction of the blood calcium below normal; manifestations include hyperactive deep tendon reflexes, muscle and abdominal cramps, and foot spasms.

**immune system** [Latin *immun*, free, exempt] This system helps protect the body from unwanted invading influences. It is the body's defense system.

**immunities** The various mechanisms of the **immune system**. There are several types (e.g., cell-mediated, **humoral**).

**immunity** The condition of being immune; security against a particular disease; nonsusceptibility to the invasive or **pathogenic** effects of foreign **microorganisms** or to the toxic effect of **antigenic** substances. The capacity to distinguish foreign material from self, and to neutralize, eliminate, or **metabolize** that which is foreign by the physiologic mechanisms of the immune response. There are several types of immunity mechanics (e.g., cell-mediated, **humoral**).

**immunoglobulins** (**Ig**) Proteins of animal origin endowed with known **antibody** activity, synthesized by lymphocytes and plasma cells. They function as specific antibodies and are responsible for the humoral aspects of immunity. They are found in the **serum** and in other body fluids and tissues, including urine, spinal fluid, lymph nodes, and spleen. There are 5 basic classes of **immunoglobulins**: IgA, IgD, IgE, IgG, and IgM.

**implantation** [Latin *in*, into + *plantare*, to set] The attachment of a **microorganism** to the lining inside the human intestine.

*in vitro* Within glass; observable in a test tube; in an artificial environment.

*in vivo* Within the living body.

**incubate** [Latin *incubare*, to lie in or on] To place in an optimal situation for development [e.g., providing the proper temperature and humidity for the growth of living cells, such as ova (eggs), microorganisms, or tissue cells].

**infection/infectious organism** Invasion and/or multiplication of **microorganisms** (the infectious organism in this case) in body tissues.

**infectious gastroenteritis** An infection pertaining to the stomach and intestines.

**infused** Filled with a certain substance or item or quality.

**insoluble** Something which cannot be dissolved into liquid form.

**intestinal commensal** An organism living on or within the intestine and deriving benefit without injuring or benefiting the host.

**intraperitoneal** Within the **peritoneal** cavity.

**Koumiss** A fermented alcoholic drink prepared from cow's milk, originally from mare's milk. Kefir koumiss is milk fermented with kefir fungi.

**kidney** Either of the two organs in the lumbar region that filter the blood, excreting the end-products of body **metabolism** in the form of urine, and regulating the concentrations of hydrogen, sodium, potassium, phosphate, and other ions in the extracellular fluid.

**klebsiella** A **genus** of **microorganisms** made up of plump, short rods with rounded ends, usually occurring singly, and frequently found in the respiratory or intestinal tract of man.

**L(+) (levorotatory)** [Latin *levo*, left + *rotare*, to turn] Turning the plane of polarized light to the left.

**L(+) lactic acid** Levorotatory **lactic acid**, or D-lactic acid, is produced by the fermentation of dextrose by micrococcus acidi levolactici. DL-lactic acid is the ordinary kind found in sour milk and certain fermented foods.

**lactase** An enzyme that helps in metabolizing lactose, also referred to as *β*-galactosidase.

**lactobacillus** (plural, **lactobacilli**) One of the six major groups of beneficial intestinal and fecal microorganisms in humans as well as animals.

**lactobacillin** A preparation of lactic acid bacteria to be added to milk to cause lactic acid fermentation.

*Lactobacillus acidophilus* (or *L. acidophilus*) A lactobacillus producing the fermented product acidophilus milk.

*L. bulgaricus* A lactobacillus producing the fermented product known as Bulgarian milk.

*Lactobacillus plantarum* Assists *L. acidophilus* in combating pathogens and has a unique ability to synthesize L-lysine.
    Lactobacillus probiotics additionally include the following:

| | |
|---|---|
| *L. salivarius* | *L. delbreucki* |
| *L. rueteri* | *L. helicticus* |
| *L. rhamnosus* | *L. casei* |
| *L. lactis* | |

**lactic acid** An acid that occurs in three forms: L, D, and DL. L is produced by **anaerobic** glycolysis in muscle during exertion. D is produced by **fermentation** of dextrose by a microorganism. DL is found in the stomach, sour milk, and certain fermented foods.

**lactic acid bacteria** (or **LAB**) These are **bacteria** that produce **lactic acid**. Lactic acid is known to exist in three forms: a dextrorotary form, L-lactic acid; a levorotatory form, D-lactic acid; a DL-lactic acid.

*L.* **var.** *rhamnosus* (var. means "variety") Same as *L. rhamnosus*.

**lactoferrin** An iron-binding protein found in some white blood cells and secretions (milk, tears, saliva, bile, etc.) displaying **bacteriocidal** activity.

**lactoperiocidase** An **enzyme** that is found in milk and saliva and is used to **catalyze** the addition of iodine to tyrosine-containing proteins.

**lactose** A sugar in milk that, when broken down, yields glucose and galactose.

**lactose intolerance** Not able to properly handle/**metabolize** **lactose**.

**lactose malabsorption** Impaired intestinal absorption of **lactose**.

**lactose tolerance test** A test for **kidney** function: 20 grams of **lactose** is dissolved in 20 ml of distilled water and injected. The urine is collected hourly and tested until the sugar reaction ceases to be positive. If lactose secretion continues for more than 5 hours, kidney disease is indicated.

**LDL** (**Low-Density** Lipoprotein) A blood plasma lipoprotein containing a low percentage of triglycerides, moderate levels of phospholipids, moderate levels of proteins, and high levels of cholesterol.

**lipase** [Greek *lipos*, fat] An **enzyme** that breaks fats (triglycerides and phospholipids) down into **fatty acids** and glycerol. These enzymes occur in milk, and in the pancreas, stomach, adipose tissue, and other tissues.

**lymphatics** This refers to the lymph vessels of the lymphatic system, often referred to as our **immune defense system**.

**lymphocyte** A type of white blood cell, part of the **immune defense system** cells of the lymph and blood circulations.

**lymphocytic** Pertaining to lymphocytes.

**macroecology** Refers to the ecology in the world around us—the outer physical world.

**macrophage** [Greek *makros*, large + *phagein*, to eat] This is a type of cell in the immune system and blood that protects us from foreign **microorganisms** and toxins, by "eating them" from our system.

**malabsorption** Impaired intestinal absorption of a substance.

**maldigestion** Improper, insufficient, or painful digestion of a substance or food.

**mammal** An animal of the type that is fed on milk produced by the mother in its infancy.

**metabolic** Pertaining to **metabolism**.

**metabolism** The sum of all the physical and chemical processes by which a living organized substance is produced and maintained (anabolism); also the transformation by which energy is made available for use by the organism (catabolism).

**metabolites** Any substance produced by metabolism or by the **metabolic** process.

**metabolize** To break down by chemical activity for use in the body.

**Metchnikoff** A Russian zoologist (1845–1916), working in Paris, who discovered phagocytes and phagocytosis.

**microbiological** [Greek *bios*, life + *mikros*, small] Pertaining to microbiology (the science which deals with the study of **microorganisms**).

**microbiota**  The microscopic living organisms of a region (e.g., in a part of the human body).

**microecology**  The ecology within our body system—the inner world.

**microorganisms**  Very small living organisms, usually microscopic. Those of medical interest are: **bacteria**, rickettsiae, viruses, molds, yeasts, and protozoa.

**miso**  A popular fermented Asian food created by aging soybeans and rice with a special starter culture. Used as a flavoring and/or a soup base.

**modulation**  The varying of the strength or nature of something.

**moiety**  [Latin *medius*, middle] A part or portion of something.

**monila vaginitis**  Monila was a former name for a **genus** of fungi now called candida. **Monila vaginitis** refers to inflammation of the vagina due or related to infection with the candida fungus.

**mutagenic**  A substance that causes or induces change and/or genetic change—mutation.

**N-nitroso compounds**  Refers to a chemical compound that contains a nitroso (N—O, nitrogen and oxygen) bond.

**nervous system**  An organ system that, along with the glandular system, correlates the adjustments and reactions of an organism to internal and environmental conditions. Includes the central nervous system (brain and spinal cord) and the peripheral nervous system (the nerves of the body, away from the central system).

**neurotransmitter**  A substance that is released at the points of impulse transmission in nerves, traveling to either excite or inhibit the target cell.

**niacin**  A water-soluble B vitamin ($B_3$) required by the body.

**nitroreductase**  An **enzyme** that adds a hydrogen atom to a substance in a reaction.

**nitrosamines**  Formed by the combination of nitrates with amines. Some nitrosamines show carcinogenic activity.

**nonessential amino acid**  An **amino acid** that is not required externally in the diet, as the body can provide it if needed.

**opportunistic**  Denoting a microorganism that does not ordinarily cause disease but which, under certain circumstances (in an impaired immune system, for instance), becomes pathogenic.

**orotic acid**  A crystalline acid that occurs in milk and is a growth factor for various **microorganisms** (as *Lactobacillus bulgaricus*).

**osteoporosis**  A condition that is characterized by decrease in bone mass with increased density and enlargement of bone spaces producing a porousness and fragileness that results from disturbances in nutrition, calcium, and mineral **metabolism**.

**oxytocin** A posterior pituitary hormone that stimulates the contraction of the uterine muscle and the secretion of milk.

**pantothenic acid** One of the B vitamins ($B_5$) that occurs in all living tissues, especially the liver. It is essential for the growth of various animals and **microorganisms**.

**pasteurized** To pasteurize is to partially sterilize a substance, especially a liquid (e.g., milk) at a temperature, and for a period of exposure, that destroys objectionable organisms.

**pathogenic** Causing, or capable of causing, disease.

**penicillin** A mixture of antibiotics produced especially by molds of the **genus** Penicillium and having a powerful **bacteriostatic** effect against various **bacteria**.

**peritoneal** The membrane lining the abdominopelvic walls and investing into the organ's cavity.

**pH** The representation of hydrogen-ion concentration of a substance: on a scale of 0 to 14 (7 represents neutral; numbers less than 7 are more acidic, have more hydrogen; numbers over 7 are more alkaline, have less hydrogen).

**phagocytes** Cells that engulf foreign material and consume debris in the normal body.

**phagocytic** Having the ability to phagocytize or function as a **phagocyte**.

**phagocytosis** The process of ingestion, isolation, and/or destruction of particulate material by **phagocytes**.

**phenolic compounds** Poisonous crystals present in coal tar and pharmaceuticals such as aspirin; regarded as a derivative of hydrocarbon.

**placque** A clear area in a bacterial **culture** produced by destruction of cells by a virus; also, an abnormal patch on a body part or surface, especially on the skin.

**plasma cell** A lymphocyte that secretes **antibodies**.

**plasmids** An extrachromosomal body other than the original **DNA** that is found in **bacteria**.

**potassium** A silvery white mineral that occurs abundantly in nature and is essential to human health. It affects the energy-requiring mechanisms within cells.

**predisposing** To bring about susceptibility to a condition or disease.

**probiotic** The beneficial, life-supporting **microorganisms** that are part of biological systems (such as the human system) and exist symbiotically with these systems.

**procarcinogens**  Substances that can promote **cancer**.

**prolactin**  A protein **hormone** of the pituitary gland that induces lactation of the breasts.

**proliferation**  Rapid and repeated production of new parts, or new growth, or of offspring (as in a mass of cells by a rapid succession of cell division).

**prophylactic**  Guarding from or preventing disease.

**propionibacterium**  A **genus** of **Gram-positive**, nonmotile **anaerobic bacteria** that form propionic acid by fermenting **lactic acid**, carbohydrates, or other substances, and that include forms associated with the ripening of dairy products.

**pseudomonas**  A **genus** of short, rod-shaped **bacteria**, many of which produce greenish fluorescent water-soluble pigment.

**psoriasis**  A chronic skin disease characterized by circumscribed red patches covered with white scales.

**putrefying**  Decomposing organic matter, typically **anaerobic** splitting of proteins by **bacteria** and fungi with the formation of foul-smelling, incompletely oxidized products.

**putrefaction**  The process of decomposition of organic matter (see **putrefying**).

**pyridoxine**  One of the B vitamins (see $B_6$).

**regimen**  A systematic plan (as of diet, therapy, or medication) often designed to improve and maintain the health of a patient.

**regularity**  The quality or state of being regular (as in bowel habits).

**resistance/resistant**  Power or capacity to resist, especially the inherent ability of an organism to resist harmful influences (a disease, toxic agents, or infections).

**reticuloendothelial system**  A system of cells spread throughout the body that functions to rid the body of debris.

**reverse osmosis**  Osmosis is the flow or diffusion that takes place through a semipermeable membrane (as of a living cell), typically separating various particles in a solution.

**salmonella**  A **genus** of **aerobic Gram-negative**, rod-shaped, non-spore-forming **bacteria** associated with various types of food poisoning and acute gastrointestinal inflammation and diseases of the genital tract.

**saturated**  A condition that means the **fatty acid** has only single bonds in its carbon chains (C—C), not double bonds (C=C).

**sedimentation**  The action or process of depositing matter that settles at the bottom of a liquid.

**sensory receptors** Nerve centers or sensitive nerves which receive sensation and communicate it to other areas of the nervous system.

**serotonin** A powerful substance that constricts veins and is found in blood serum and in the gastric (stomach) mucosa of mammals.

**serum** The clear yellowish fluid that remains after suspended material (such as blood cells), fibrinogen, and fibrin (the clotting substances in blood) are removed.

**sex hormones** **Hormones** (from the gonads or adrenal cortex) that affect the growth or function of the reproductive organs or the development of secondary sex characteristics.

**shigella** A **genus** of nonmotile **aerobic** **bacteria** that form acid but no gas on many carbohydrates and that cause **dysentery** in animals—especially in humans.

**short generation time** A very short period of time between the production of each next generation of cells in a bacterial culture.

**short lag-phase** A short space of time between phenomena or related events.

**soluble** Existing in a state that renders a substance susceptible to being dissolved in a fluid.

**solute** A dissolved substance, especially a component of a solution present in smaller amounts than the fluid.

**sonicate** To disrupt **bacteria** cells by treatment with high-frequency sound waves.

**spasm** A constriction of a passageway, or an involuntary contraction of muscle, attended by pain and loss of function, producing abnormal movement and distortion.

**species** A category of biological classification ranking immediately below the **genus** or subgenus, comprising related organisms or populations potentially capable of interbreeding.

**specificity** The condition of being peculiar to a particular individual or group of organisms; also, the condition of participating in or catalyzing only one or a few chemical reactions.

**spectrum** A range of effectiveness against **pathogenic** organisms (e.g., an antibiotic with a broad spectrum).

**stability** The quality, state, or degree of being stable, not changing or fluctuating, or of being readily altered in chemical or physical makeup.

**staphylococcus** A **genus** of nonmotile, **Gram-positive**, spherical **bacteria** of the skin and mucus membranes.

**sterile** Free from living organisms and especially **microorganisms**.

**steroid hormones** Any of numerous **hormones** (e.g., the sex hormones, cortisone, adrenocortical hormones) having the characteristic ring structure of steroids.

**strain** A group of presumed common ancestry with clear-cut physiological, but usually not morphological (shape), distinctions.

**streptococcus** A **genus** of nonmotile, chiefly parasitic, **Gram-positive bacteria**; some are pathogens of man and domestic animals.

*Streptococcus thermophilus* A Gram-positive microorganism that is used along with *Lactobacillus bulgaricus* to make yogurt.

**streptomycin** An **antibiotic** used especially in the treatment of infections (e.g., tuberculosis) by **Gram-negative bacteria**.

**subspecies** A subdivision of a **species**.

**supernatant** Usually a clear liquid overlying material deposited by settling, precipitation, or **centrifugation**.

**suppression** Stoppage of a bodily function or a symptom, the failure of development, or the inhibiting of a genetic expression (e.g., **suppression** of a mutation).

**synergism** Interaction of separate agents or substances such that the total effect is greater than the sum of individual effects.

**synergistically** Having the capacity to act in **synergism**.

**terrain** An area of land or an area of tissue in the body with regard to its natural makeup or characteristics.

**toxins** A colloidal protein-type poisonous substance that is a specific product of the metabolic activities of a living organism and is usually very unstable, notably toxic when introduced into the tissues, and typically capable of inducing antibody formation.

**transient** Lasting only for a short time; quickly passing.

**tryptophan** An **amino acid** that is widely distributed in proteins and is essential to animal life.

**tumor** An abnormal mass of tissue that is not inflammatory, arises from cells of preexistent tissue, and serves no useful purpose.

**tyrosine** A **metabolically** important **amino acid**.

**ultrafiltration** Filtration through a medium that allows small molecules to pass but holds back larger ones (as protein does).

**umeboshi plums** Salt-pickled plums from the Prunis mume tree used in Japanese cooking.

**urea** The chief nitrogen end-product of the **metabolism** of proteins. It is formed in the liver from **amino acids** and from compounds of ammonia.

**urinary indican** Formed by the decomposition of **tryptophan** in the intestines and then excreted in the urine.

**urinary tract** The channel through which urine passes and which consists of the renal tubules, pelvis of the **kidney**, ureters, bladder, and urethra.

**uropathogens** **Microorganisms** that cause diseases of the **urinary tract**.

**vaginitis** Inflammation of the vagina, often with itching irritation.

**viability** The capacity or capability of living.

**viable** Capable of living.

**virulent** Able to overcome bodily defense mechanisms, marked by a rapid, severe, and fatal course.

**vitamin K** A fat-soluble vitamin, essential for clotting of the blood.

**vulvovaginitis** Inflammation of the vulva and vagina.

**whey** The serum or watery part of milk that is separated from the curd part. It is rich in **lactose**, minerals, and vitamins, and has traces of fat.

**yogurt** A fermented, slightly acid, often flavored, semisolid food made of whole or skimmed cow's milk and milk solids to which **cultures** of **bacteria** of the **genus** *L. bulgaricus* and *S. thermophilus* have been added.

# Index

**143**

# ABOUT THE AUTHORS

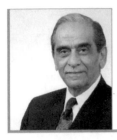

## Khem M. Shahani, Ph.D.

Widely regarded as one of the world's leading research authorities on the role of lactobacilli and gastrointestinal bacteria in human nutrition and health, Dr. Khem Shahani has published more than 200 peer-reviewed scientific articles related to microorganisms and health.

Earning his Masters in Biochemistry in his native India, Dr. Shahani then earned his doctorate, specializing in dairy foods technology, nutrition, microbiology, and biochemistry—the predeterminants of Biotechnology—at the University of Wisconsin. He worked at both the University of Illinois and Ohio State University before accepting tenure with the Department of Dairy Sciences and the Department of Food Science and Technology at the University of Nebraska.

At the University of Nebraska, research on *Lactobacillus acidophilus* was started as early as 1925—over 70 years ago. For over 40 years, scientists headed by Dr. Shahani worked on *Lactobacillus acidophilus*, yogurt cultures (*Lactobacillus bulgaricus* and *Streptococcus thermophilus*), *Lactobacillus bifidus* (now renamed *Bifidobacterium bifidum*) and other lactic cultures. Dr. Shahani began these endeavors when he saw that getting the benefits of these flora from both foods and supplements was difficult at best. He felt compelled to find the best strains (varieties of microorganisms within species, characterized by their particular qualities) as well as new and superior growth and preservation techniques to ensure successful colonization of beneficial flora in the body.

His work addressed the most critical issues: stability, viability, and bioactivity of the flora cells; resistance to digestive acidity; antibiotic and probiotic aspects; and, above all, successful probiotic implementation in the human system. In addition, he developed an unsurpassed stabilization process for the beneficial bacteria.

During his tenure, Dr. Shahani isolated, developed, and optimized exceptional strains of microorganisms, the most noted of which is a particular strain of *Lactobacillus acidophilus* that has become internationally acclaimed as the DDS-1 (Department of Dairy Sciences Number 1) strain. Often regarded as the "Cadillac" of the *L. acidophilus* class of probiotics, DDS-1 is currently distributed worldwide. Unquestionably producing the finest flora, Dr. Shahani's special production methods are exclusive, and his strains are among only a few to be produced at a university research facility.

In addition to his work at the University of Nebraska, his expertise on milk, yogurt, and the dairy industry, made him a leading consultant for the Food Industry. Dr. Shahani also founded and served as the Scientific Director of Nebraska Cultures, Inc. (now based in Walnut Creek, California), where he developed strains and cultures of friendly flora for use as dietary supplements. As a consultant to several food-supplement manufacturing organizations and to governments worldwide, as well as international groups such as the World Health Organization (WHO) of the United Nations, Dr. Shahani received numerous awards for scientific achievement and service. It is no wonder Dr. Shahani has often been cited as "the mastermind" behind today's currently thriving and expanding probiotic industry worldwide.

# Betsy F. Meshbesher, D.C.

Betsy F. Meshbesher, D.C., has been working in the nutritional field for 27 years. Internationally regarded as one of the most well-versed researchers on the specialty subject of natural versus synthetic nutrition, Dr. Meshbesher devotes much of her time researching, writing, lecturing, and helping other health professionals successfully implement clinical nutrition into their practices. She has also served as a technical advisor and consultant to several major nutrition companies.

Dr. Meshbesher completed her undergraduate work at the University of Minnesota and earned her doctorate degree at Northwestern College of Chiropractic in 1986. A protégé to Dr. Richard Murray, she is also recognized as the most outstanding student of Dr. Royal Lee (of Standard Process Vitamins), considered by many to have been the best-informed nutritionist of his time.

Well known for her research and development of *The Bodymaker*™ Cleanse and Digestive System Rehabilitation Program, Dr. Meshbesher currently serves as Executive Director of Meshbesher Health Corporation. This corporation provides health professionals with the products and services needed to attain flourishing nutritional practices. She is also the founder of Biotrophic Nutrients Corporation, which features a full line of natural whole-food-concentrate nutritionals.

# Venkat Mangalampalli, Ph.D.

Venkat Mangalampalli has a Ph.D. in Biochemistry from India and has worked in several capacities in renowned pharmaceutical R&D laboratories in India. For the past 10 years, he has been working in the area of food science and technology. His specialization includes the development of a process for combining microbial metabolites and functional foods with probiotics, phytonutrients, and enzymes for therapeutic use. He has published 20 scientific papers in the areas of process development and functional foods. He worked as a postdoctoral research associate with Dr. Shahani at the Department of Food Science and Technology, University of Nebraska–Lincoln, from 1998 to 2000. He is currently working in the pharmaceutical industry.

# Resources

**Solaray**
Multidophilus Plus DDS-1
(capsules/chewable)

**TwinLab**
Super Acidophilus

**Roex Products**
Colon Essentials

**Biotics Research**
Biodophilus

RECOMMENDED PROBIOTIC SUPPLEMENTS AVAILABLE BY DIRECT ORDER

**Arise and Shine**
www.ariseandshine.com
Flora Grow
Yeast End

**American Biologics**
1180 Walnut Ave.
Chula Vista, CA 91911
800-227-4458
www.americanbiologics.com
Bio-Dophilus Capsules
Bio-Bifidus Powder
Ultra Microplex Powder

**Dr. Shahani's Probiotics**
www..drshahani.com
*Lactobacillus acidophilus* DDS-1 and
other probiotic formulas

**Optimal Health Systems**
222 West Center St.
Pima, AZ 85543
800-890-4547
www.optimalhealthsystems.com
Opti-Cleanse
Optimal Defense

**Nutratec** (Italy)
+39 0722 327 573
www.nutratec.it
DDS-1 *L. acidophilus*

**AnnCare** (Taiwan)
www.anncare.com
DDS-1 (powder)
DDS-1 (capsules)

**Natural Wellness Centers**
www.naturalwellness.com
Pro-Biotics Plus (capsules/chewable)

FOOD SOURCES OF PROBIOTICS AVAILABLE IN HEALTH FOOD STORES

Organic yogurt and kefirs (with live
active probiotic cultures):
**Seven Stars**
**Horizon**
**Brown Cow**
**Stonyfield Farm**
**Helios Nutrition's Kefir**
  (with FOS/inulin)
**Lifeway Kefir**
**Windhaven Sheep Yoghurt**
  (not certified)

**Meyenberg Goat Milk Products**
  (not certified)
AU: **Barambah Organics**
NZ: **BioFarm Yoghurt**
UK: **Rachel's Organics**
  **Yeo Valley**

Nondairy:
**Cascadian Farm Organic Sauerkraut**
**Eden Organic Sauerkraut**
**Deep Root** (organic cultured
  vegetables)

RECOMMENDED READING

*The Yeast Connection,* William G. Crook (Vintage)

*Candida and M.E. (Fibromyalgia)* (WDDTY Publications)

*Trace Your Genes to Health* (yeast-inhibiting diet), Chris Reading, M.D. (Vital Health Publishing)

*The No Grain Diet,* Dr. Joseph Mercola (Dutton)

*The Body Ecology Diet,* Donna Gates (Body Ecology)

*Stomach Ailments and Digestive Disturbances,* Michael T. Murray, ND

MORE INFORMATION ON PROBIOTICS, INTESTINAL BALANCE, AND THE EFFECTS OF ANTIBIOTIC USE

**Nebraska Cultures**, Inc.
Information on probiotics, digestive health, and the DDS-1 strain of *Lactobacillus acidophilus*
1911 Trenton Court
Walnut Creek, CA 94596
925-935-0922
www.nebraskacultures.com

**The Cure Zone** Web site
"Educating Instead of Medicating"
www.curezone.com

**What Doctor's Don't Tell You**
A searchable Web site of the past 15 years of research from the respected independent medical journal *What Doctor's Don't Tell You*
www.wddty.com

LABORATORIES THAT TEST FOR INTESTINAL DYSBIOSIS

**AAL Reference Laboratories, Inc.**
1715 E. Wilshire #715
Santa Ana, CA 92705
(714) 972-9979
(800) 522-2611
(714) 543-2034 FAX
www.antibodyassay.com

**Great Smokies Diagnostic Laboratory**
63 Zillicoa Street
Asheville, NC 28801-1074
(704) 253-0621
(800) 522-4762
Email: cs@gsdl.com
www.gsdl.com

**Immuno Laboratories, Inc.**
1620 W. Oakland Park Blvd.
Ft. Lauderdale, FL 33311
(305) 486-4500
(800) 231-9197
(305) 739-6563 (fax)
Email: info@immunolabs.com
www.immunolabs.com

**Immunosciences Lab, Inc.**
8730 Wilshire Blvd., Suite 305
Beverly Hills, CA 90211
(310) 657-1077
(800) 950-4686
(310) 657-1053 FAX
Email: immunsci@ix.netcom.com
www.immuno-sci-lab.com

ALTERNATIVE PHYSICIAN SOURCES

**The American College for Advancement in Medicine**
1-888-439-6891
www.acam.org
This organization has a Web site and call center that helps you locate an alternative physician.

**Health World Online**
The oldest, established health-information site on the Web, Health World lets you search all of the major accredited alternative health associations in the United States to find a practitioner, or to find news articles, related books, and columns by leading practitioners.
www.healthy.net/

**The International Health Foundation**
The president of this organization and author of *The Yeast Connection*, Dr. William Crook, maintains a list of doctors who treat the condition. You may contact the foundation for a referral at:
The International Health Foundation
P.O. Box 3494
Jackson, TN 38303
901-660-7090

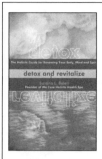
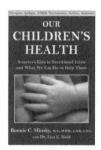
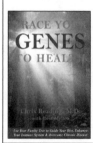